Evaluating Health Promotion Programs

Marc T. Braverman, *Editor*
University of California, Davis

NEW DIRECTIONS FOR PROGRAM EVALUATION

A Publication of the American Evaluation Association

A joint organization of the Evaluation Research Society and the Evaluation Network

NICK L. SMITH, *Editor-in-Chief*
Syracuse University

Number 43, Fall 1989

Paperback sourcebooks in
The Jossey-Bass Higher Education
and Social and Behavioral Science Series

Jossey-Bass Inc., Publishers
San Francisco • Oxford

Marc T. Braverman (ed.).
Evaluating Health Promotion Programs.
New Directions for Program Evaluation, no. 43.
San Francisco: Jossey-Bass, 1989.

New Directions for Program Evaluation Series
A publication of the American Evaluation Association
Nick L. Smith, *Editor-in-Chief*

New Directions for Program Evaluation is published quarterly by
Jossey-Bass Inc., Publishers (publication number USPS 449-050),
and is sponsored by the American Evaluation Association.
Second-class postage rates are paid at San Francisco, California,
and at additional mailing offices. POSTMASTER: Send address
changes to Jossey-Bass Inc., Publishers, 350 Sansome Street,
San Francisco, California 94104.

Editorial correspondence should be sent to the Editor-in-Chief,
Nick L. Smith, School of Education, Syracuse University,
330 Huntington Hall, Syracuse, N.Y. 13244-2340.

Library of Congress Catalog Card Number LC 85-644749

International Standard Serial Number ISSN 0164-7989

International Standard Book Number ISBN 1-55542-854-1

Cover art by WILLI BAUM

Manufactured in the United States of America. Printed on acid-free paper.

Ordering Information

The paperback sourcebooks listed below are published quarterly and can be ordered either by subscription or single copy.

Subscriptions cost $64.00 per year for institutions, agencies, and libraries. Individuals can subscribe at the special rate of $48.00 per year *if payment is by personal check.* (Note that the full rate of $64.00 applies if payment is by institutional check, even if the subscription is designated for an individual.) Standing orders are accepted.

Single copies are available at $14.95 when payment accompanies order. (California, New Jersey, New York, and Washington, D.C., residents please include appropriate sales tax.) For billed orders, cost per copy is $14.95 plus postage and handling.

Substantial discounts are offered to organizations and individuals wishing to purchase bulk quantities of Jossey-Bass sourcebooks. Please inquire.

Please note that these prices are for the calendar year 1989 and are subject to change without prior notice. Also, some titles may be out of print and therefore not available for sale.

To ensure correct and prompt delivery, all orders must give either the *name of an individual* or an *official purchase order number.* Please submit your order as follows:

Subscriptions: specify series and year subscription is to begin.
Single Copies: specify sourcebook code (such as, PE1) and first two words of title.

Mail all orders to:
Jossey-Bass Inc., Publishers
350 Sansome Street
San Francisco, California 94104

New Directions for Program Evaluation Series
Nick L. Smith, *Editor-in-Chief*

New Directions for Program Evaluation

Sponsored by the American Evaluation Association
(A Joint Organization of the Evaluation Research Society
and the Evaluation Network)

American Evaluation Association, 9555 Persimmon Tree Road, Potomac, MD 20854

Contents

The difficulties in evaluating media-based health promotion programs are described, and two evaluation designs are proposed for media campaigns.

These proposed guidelines for reports of health program evaluations bring to light several critical issues related to the interpretability of studies.

Editor's Notes

Health promotion programs aim to shape individual behavior and other factors that affect our society's collective health. Such programs have jumped to the forefront of the nation's consciousness in the past decade. Taken as a whole, these programs constitute an extremely important and rapidly expanding area for evaluation research and practice.

The growth of health promotion programming can be attributed to a convergence of several factors. First is the message from public health scientists that the greatest health threats facing us today—cancer, AIDS, cardiovascular disease, lung and liver disorders, and automobile injuries, to name but a few—are strongly linked to behavior and lifestyle, to a far greater degree than were the infectious diseases that threatened previous generations. Second is the high cost of sickness, in terms of both lives and money, and the difficulties encountered in research on treatments. A third factor is the emergence of several highly volatile social issues, such as illegal drug use, nonsmokers' rights, and alcohol-related automobile injuries, that have galvanized communities and spurred grass-roots efforts to seek solutions. All of these factors have combined to support prevention, largely in the form of social programs, as an essential adjunct to the treatment of disease and injury. The federal government has been an active partner in this movement, as evidenced most clearly by the release in 1979 of *Healthy People: The Surgeon General's Report on Health Promotion and Disease Prevention,* which led to the formulation of 226 national health objectives targeted for the year 1990. The development of health objectives for the year 2000 is currently under way at the U.S. Public Health Service.

The programs that have emerged tackle their respective issues in a variety of settings, including schools, communities, worksites, and mass communication channels. The scope of programs ranges from national initiatives to storefront operations. Outcomes are frequently elusive, the supporting theory changes rapidly, outside interest is intense, and methodological or ethical problems may be substantial. Into this picture the program evaluator must step, to play a leadership role in clarifying debates, setting standards, and developing mechanisms for learning about these programs.

The intent of this volume is to provide a number of perspectives that

I would like to thank Joel M. Moskowitz, Carol N. D'Onofrio, and Jana Kay Slater for their invaluable assistance in the preparation of this volume. Their comments and insights were much appreciated.

1

can help evaluators fulfill these crucial functions. Several of the chapters discuss conceptual themes of program theory and context, whereas other chapters cover important topics related to measurement, data analysis, and research design. The final chapter discusses the reporting of evaluation studies. Considered together, the chapters present several of the most critical issues in a framework intended to inform and support evaluations of health promotion programs.

In Chapter One, Donald T. Campbell and I address the political and social context in which many health programs are delivered and evaluated. External pressures may conflict with the atmosphere of unbiased analysis and self-criticism needed for honest program evaluation efforts. The chapter discusses nonscientific imperatives and their social science implications and provides recommendations for evaluators and program sponsors.

In Chapter Two, Christine Jackson, David G. Altman, Beth Howard-Pitney, and John W. Farquhar analyze issues related to community-based health interventions. These are often among the most complex of programs, entailing multiple components and audiences. In covering such topics as program and audience definition, the ethics of program delivery, and the role of community stakeholders, the authors provide an analysis with broad applicability for evaluators and program planners.

For health promotion programs, the determination of appropriate outcomes—the expectations about program success—may be very complex. As J. Allan Best and his colleagues describe in Chapter Three, the evaluator often must hypothesize precursors of behavioral change, designate appropriate timeframes, and address change at both the individual and system levels. The authors challenge several traditional approaches to outcome formulation and present a multidimensional model for use in the definition of outcomes.

Frederica W. O'Connor, Thomas D. Cook, and Elizabeth C. Devine treat health program implementation issues in Chapter Four. Describing a case study of a hospital-based patient education program, they review the contributions of meta-analysis, theory, and site-specific knowledge to the design of an implementation strategy. The authors also describe the process of developing measures and the use of a critical multiplism approach in the interpretation of results.

One of the most significant modes of data collection for health program evaluations is the use of participants' self-reports, and this mode is examined by Carol N. D'Onofrio in Chapter Five. In many cases, the self-report format is indispensable for gaining information about such sensitive behaviors as drug and alcohol use or sexual practices. D'Onofrio analyzes possible sources of reporting bias and analyzes ethical and validity issues in the use of self-report measures.

David Koepke and Brian R. Flay, in Chapter Six, address issues related to the evaluation unit, a complex series of considerations well known to many program evaluators. The authors' coverage is both theoretical and practical and includes recommendations for improving the accuracy of research design and analysis.

Jack McKillip, in Chapter Seven, addresses the use of media campaigns to promote health. He discusses the difficulties inherent in implementing standard designs for evaluating media-based programs, and he offers two quasi-experimental designs that use multiple measurements on a single population to determine no-treatment baselines.

Joel M. Moskowitz, in Chapter Eight, considers what needs to be known about a program and its evaluation before one can adequately understand its implementation and results. He suggests guidelines for reporting health program evaluations, and these guidelines should stimulate thinking and discussion on possible standards in this area. The interpretability issues that Moskowitz addresses are related to such topics as program theory, program delivery, sampling, attrition, and statistical power.

These chapters provide a discussion of some of the most important issues confronting the evaluation of health promotion programs. This volume is intended both to facilitate debate on these issues and to provide guidance for those who face the very real demands of program evaluation. Ultimately, we hope this work will contribute to improved programming and better health for our communities.

Marc T. Braverman
Editor

Marc T. Braverman is educational research and evaluation specialist for the University of California Cooperative Extension/4-H and a faculty member in human development at the University of California, Davis.

Research on health promotion programming often functions under substantial external pressures, which can complicate the research enterprise.

Facilitating the Development of Health Promotion Programs: Recommendations for Researchers and Funders

Marc T. Braverman, Donald T. Campbell

Protecting the nation's health through the promotion of desirable behavioral lifestyles is a strategy of high priority for national policymakers and the public health community. This theme is clearly visible, for instance, in the Public Health Service's national health objectives for the year 1990 (U.S. Department of Health and Human Services, 1986), which call for preventive education efforts in the areas of drug and alcohol abuse, smoking, sexually transmitted diseases, infant health, control of obesity and eating disorders, teenage pregnancy, and other health concerns. Many stakeholder groups have high expectations for these programs to effect behavioral change at the individual level, with consequent improvements in large-scale health promotion and disease prevention.

The rapid proliferation of health promotion programs has far outpaced the deliberative attempts of social scientists to determine their effectiveness. Efforts to pull together the accumulating research base are exceedingly difficult. Furthermore, the emphasis placed on program evaluation is uneven. Depending on the funding agency, in many cases it

Marc T. Braverman (ed.). *Evaluating Health Promotion Programs.*
New Directions for Program Evaluation, no. 43. San Francisco: Jossey-Bass, Fall 1989.

is not required at all (General Accounting Office, 1987; Morrison and Sivilli, 1987). In other cases, the urgency of the debates in the public and legislative sectors and the instability of the funding have often introduced extreme pressures for "effective" programs to be developed and disseminated over a very short time. Social scientists are well aware that these pressures come into conflict with the way information on program effectiveness is gained.

Within this context, much more attention needs to be given to the validity of the social science enterprise itself, as affected by the organizational structures and processes whereby knowledge claims are generated and shared among researchers, funders, and other stakeholders. This chapter is a step in that direction, drawing on previous work related to the sociology of scientific validity (Campbell, 1984, 1986b, 1987). Our primary focus is on sponsored research involving primary prevention education for youth.

The discussion has two major sections. In the first, we note several characteristics of the current environment for research and evaluation related to health promotion programs. In the second, we list several recommendations for the organization and focus of research activity. Our analysis and recommendations are offered in the spirit of the following overriding goals:

- To increase coordination within the research community working in health promotion, particularly through mechanisms of mutual reinforcement and monitoring
- To strengthen the empirical base from which researchers can build on one another's work
- To maintain rigor in the face of strong pressures for "effective" panaceas
- To acknowledge and respond to pressures from outside communities, to the extent that this is possible without jeopardizing scientific validity.

Our arguments will be illustrated with examples drawn primarily from the prevention of drug and tobacco use. Both areas encompass a range of educational approaches that provide a good historical perspective for considering the growth of programmatic understanding. Drug abuse, in particular, is arguably the behavioral health topic that stirs the highest degree of passion in public debate, receiving an uninterrupted stream of attention from lawmakers, journalists, and assorted social critics.

Characteristics of the Current Environment for Health Promotion Research

First of all, there is a wide perception that education, if only it is provided with enough funding, can have strong and/or immediate impacts on health problems. The past ten years have witnessed an upsurge of interest in the use of educational programming for achieving health objectives. In many specific areas this is largely due to disillusion with previous emphases. For example, interest in smoking prevention has risen in proportion to despair over the rate of progress in cancer treatment. In the case of drug abuse, interest in educational approaches is tied to the growing acknowledgment of the failure to control drug abuse through interdiction and law enforcement efforts.

The contrast in views on the potential of school-based programs to solve (or begin to solve) the illegal drug problem is well illustrated by several excerpts from the 1986 hearings before the House of Representatives' Select Committee on Narcotics Abuse and Control. The transcripts reveal these quotes from legislators (U.S. Congress, 1987):

> *Congressman B. Gilman:* Drug abuse has swept across our nation's schools with a fervor rarely matched, and while the law enforcement community battles the narcotics traffickers with every tool at their disposal, it is clear that this rising tide cannot be stemmed unless and until we place a comprehensive emphasis on the dire need for drug abuse education [Part II, p. 25].

> *Congressman J. Wright:* With drug use reaching epidemic levels in our schools, anti-drug education is the only really effective antidote. . . . Education can give students the knowledge and skills they need to resist a dangerous threat to their own lives and their own futures [Part I, p. 51].

Contrasted to the remarks of the congressmen are the more circumspect comments of then-secretary of education William Bennett:

> What we want at the Department of Education is to get drugs out of school—right now, no ifs, ands, or buts. We think it is critical to get them out. If there is a set of packaged material, curriculum material, that will assure us we will get drugs out, we will buy it and distribute it where it should be distributed. We have seen no such set of materials yet. We are strongly in favor of drug education programs, but I have to point out, Mr. Chairman, whether mandated or not, almost every school district in this country has drug education programs, and we are still awash in drugs [Part I, p. 23].

With increasing frequency, researchers are beginning to question the degree to which education per se, in its narrow definition as program packages delivered in schools, can be effective in reducing the use of harmful substances. The research community is turning toward a broader interpretation of the causes of substance abuse, one that reduces the

8

potency of educational intervention—considered in isolation—to serve as a change agent. Many researchers (Goodstadt, 1987; Wallack and Corbett, 1987), as well as some policymakers (Pollin, 1987) and educators (U.S. Department of Education, 1986), propose that substantial change cannot occur without simultaneous action on the social environment that sanctions such behavior (including the microenvironment of the child), whether the substance in question is tobacco, alcohol, or an illegal drug. Thus, this position advocates the coordinated use of educational, environmental, and regulatory initiatives, rather than narrow reliance on the educational option alone.

Second, the growth of understanding about program effectiveness is a slow process. This point is well illustrated by the development of program theory in smoking prevention (Best and others, 1988; Janicki and Braverman, 1986), drug abuse prevention (Klitzner, 1987; Tobler, 1986), alcohol abuse prevention (Moskowitz, 1989), and almost any other health promotion area. Theory development progresses, not in smooth increments, but fitfully through shifts in research perspectives and themes. Smoking prevention, for example, has seen emphasis on straight information presentation, comprehensive life skills, and psychosocial influences, among other themes.

One issue related to the development of programmatic theory is the distortion of theoretical concepts that sometimes results from the translation of program ideas into popular conceptions. For example, Evans's (1988) comments regarding the "Say No to Drugs" campaign illustrate the problems inherent in isolating program subelements. "Just say no" has become a public and political rallying point, and one can argue that the prevailing public perception of drug education consists simply of convincing youth to follow this maxim. However, the psychological theme that underlies this campaign—the concept of social refusal skills in the face of direct peer pressure—is only one component of social influences-based substance abuse prevention programs. One can reasonably assume that all researchers working in preventive education recognize that the reasons youth begin to experiment with illegal drugs, tobacco, or alcohol are varied and complex, encompassing issues of self-definition, autonomy, social modeling, risk taking, and values formation (to name just a few), in addition to direct peer pressure. Evans asserts that the elevation of this single strategic component into an overall public relations theme is in fact an incorrect and perhaps even counterproductive oversimplification. This example illustrates the dangers of extrapolating single program elements into context-free beliefs about causality. It also illustrates how the public, when faced with a perceived urgent need for information, may take limited program information and reinterpret it into overly reductive terms. The problem is really one of external validity: determining how the results of one or more studies can be applied to different settings and audiences. Social scientists need to be acutely aware of the validity implications of their research and may need to be more active in discussing this issue with policymakers.

Third, coordination within the social science community is low; funding support and use of evaluation are erratic. The field of drug education provides the most striking illustration of this point. Morrison and Sivilli (1987) found that as of mid 1987, at the federal level alone, there were sixty-five drug education or prevention programs being administered by eight federal agencies, including ACTION and the Departments of Defense, Education, Health and Human Services, Interior, Justice, Transportation, and Treasury. Within these agencies the splintering effect was also strongly present. Coordination of these programs is a massive task, one that the federal government so far has not been able to accomplish adequately (U.S. Department of Education, 1987).

Another characteristic of federal-level support for research and development is unstable funding. Past patterns show short-lived legislative interest. This situation leads to a strong sense of caution in the research community in response to sudden funding initiatives for drug education (Bales, 1987). One consequence of the rapid shifts in funding support is that it has been difficult to build provisions for long-term follow-up into research planning.

Most programs are delivered without sufficient evaluation of their effects. At the federal level, Morrison and Sivilli (1987) found that few projects reported ongoing or planned evaluations. Many of those that did report evaluation activity operationalized it simply as project monitoring or as keeping track of participation counts (number of activities held, number of persons in attendance, and so forth). Impact evaluations were rare.

At the state level the situation is much the same, as evidenced by a survey of state alcohol and drug abuse agencies regarding the nature and extent of educational programming for students (U.S. Department of Education, 1987). When asked to identify the bases of their judgments on program effectiveness, 93 percent of state administrators responded "professional judgment," while only 22 percent responded "formal evaluation" and 9 percent responded "district records." These state officials appear to have been making their judgments of empirical effectiveness primarily on the basis of nonempirical processes.

Thus, it is very difficult to take stock of the current status and impact of preventive education in schools. From the standpoint of social science, this represents a lost opportunity of major proportions. The wide scope of delivery settings presents the possibility for cross-validating a range of procedures and program approaches.

Fourth, policymakers desire immediate, favorable (if possible), and at least unambiguous evaluation information. Our citations from the transcripts of the congressional hearings underscore the frequent desire of legislators and policymakers for immediate, unambiguous information on which programs work and which ones do not. Evaluators are well aware of ambiguities in their findings, of plausible rival explanations, of measurement compromises, of problems in trying to generalize to other program settings, and so forth. In large part, policymakers are not fully aware of these considerations and are frustrated by the many qualifications needed in interpretation. Thus, one characteristically strong demand with respect to communication between researchers and practitioners is absence of complication. In statistical terms, this expectation could be described as one of highly dependable and simple main-effect relationships between independent (program) and dependent (outcome) variables. Yet we know that in social science such relationships are rare (Campbell, 1986a).

A case in point is the U.S. Department of Education's (1986) pamphlet entitled *What Works: Schools Without Drugs.* The pamphlet is written in a confident, authoritative tone that stands in sharp contrast to the cautious and messy conclusions one finds in published research articles. In its opening pages it states, "[This pamphlet] provides a practical synthesis of the most reliable and significant findings available on drug use by school-age youth. It tells how extensive drug use is and how dangerous it is. It tells how drug use starts, how it progresses, and how it can be identified. *Most important, it tells how it can be stopped.* It recommends strategies—and describes particular communities—that have succeeded in beating drugs" (page v; emphasis in original). While the recommendations appear fundamentally sound within the limits of present findings—particularly the attention to such environmental issues as school policies and school-community partnerships—we feel that the definitiveness with which the recommendations are presented is overstated. The explicit curriculum recommendations betray no sense of equivocal findings or differential effectiveness of various strategies across subpopulations of youth, nor, in general, do the recommendations convey that the body of knowledge about drug program effectiveness is still very much in transition. Indeed, the pamphlet can be seen to illustrate an approach to "what works" in the communication of research results to administrators and practitioners.

Sometimes a very strong and effective program, introduced with no thought of evaluation, nevertheless produces such clear-cut effects that convincing retrospective evaluations are possible. Our methodological literature becomes misleading by featuring such illustrations. Thus, striking graphs from Aschenfelter's job-training study and the British breathalyzer crackdown are widely displayed (Cook and Campbell, 1979, pp. 219, 229; Campbell, 1988). This situation is far from the case in the present arena, where the uncoordinated multiplicity of programs means that potential comparison or control groups are apt to be treated by alternative programs. In addition, most of the programs are under-budgeted tokens, too weak to leave any clear shadow on the available records.

Recommendations for Research and Program Development

The following recommendations are geared toward developing a mutually reinforcing applied social science community working in the area of health promotion. The recommendations follow generally from Campbell's (1984, 1986b) previous work on the sociology of scientific validity, and they build particularly on a set of guidelines developed for the management of mental health research (Campbell, 1987). Recommendations 1 through 5, which involve evaluative validity, are relevant to all research and development in the area of health promotion. Recommendations 6 through 10, which involve the organization of research activities, are relevant primarily to research projects funded through grants from governmental agencies or private foundations.

1. Validity of treatments. In any field trial of a health promotion program, the primary concern should be its *local molar validity*, by which we mean attention to the program as a global entity. This view can be characterized by the question "Did this complex treatment package make a real difference in this unique application at this particular place and time?" (Campbell, 1986a). One reason for this position is that it is impossible to establish, with a high degree of confidence, any relation-ship between a single program element and its educational outcome when these are taken out of their programmatic context (Cook, 1985). These relationships, studied "in vitro" so to speak, must necessarily demand a lower level of confidence than exists for the study as a whole, for which all the original decisions involving sampling, assignment, implementation, personnel, and so forth, apply. The "Just say no" movement, discussed above, is one example of the misinterpretations that may occur.

2. Generalization to other settings. The question of whether one can generalize the outcomes of a single program field trial to other persons, settings, or times—leaving constant the treatment itself and the measures employed in the evaluation—may best be addressed, not through large-scale representative sampling, but through atheoretical judgments made on the basis of clinical experience, experimental results, the predictions of formal theory, and so forth. This principle of *proximal similarity* (Campbell, 1986a) for judging generalizability is probably better suited to social science research than is a strict dependence on statistical sampling. Past experience in social science shows that higher-order interactions are much more common than are easily interpretable main-effect relationships between independent and dependent variables. This causes considerable complications for generalizing purely on the basis of statistical reasoning.

3. Wider use of formative evaluation in project development. Funders of health programs tend to place heavy emphasis on the evaluation of program impacts, an emphasis stemming in large part from their preference for unambiguous, readily usable results. From their perspective, this emphasis is justifiable, but it should not dissuade researchers from devoting the time, attention, and resources needed for formative evaluation during a project's developmental stages. These more informal evaluation processes are typically applied to a host of programmatic decisions—for example, determining the optimal sequence for a series of curriculum sessions or the contents of a training day for prospective program leaders. Clearly, these decisions, considered in their aggregate, can have enormous implications for a program's eventual success, and yet one obviously cannot construct an experiment to test each one. The informal but systematic kinds of information gathering that precede these decisions should be conducted in full awareness of the underlying causal inferences and available decision options. Toward that end, each project researcher should keep a record or log that details the project's formative evaluation processes in weighing such decision options.

The timing and coordination of formative and impact evaluation activities is an essential consideration. In health promotion programming, there is frequently a rush to subject immature programs to summative evaluation before they have been developed to a point of treatment integrity and stability. Because such haste can lead to serious misjudgments about programs, it should be avoided, despite sometimes strong pressures for a finished product. In this context, formative evaluation techniques deserve much longer utilization timetables.

4. Monitoring of treatment delivery in experimental and comparison groups. It has become fairly well accepted in intervention research that the fidelity of treatment delivery, and the reactions of treatment recipients, need to be assessed (see McCaul and Glasgow, 1985). Often, however, this attention applies only to the experimental treatments, while the assumption is made that the comparison group got no treatment and required no monitoring during the study. On the contrary, it is very important to monitor the activities of the comparison group and the perceptions of the comparison subjects. Health interventions are sufficiently commonplace that members of experimental as well as comparison groups may be receiving similar programs from other sources. Indeed, this well may be the norm rather than the exception in prevention programs for adolescents. Knowledge of the nature and extent of these programs and of the subjects who are exposed to them is essential to correct interpretation of experimental results.

5. *The role of qualitative knowing in interpreting results.* By the term *qualitative knowing*, we refer to situation-specific knowledge about the course of events in any given study. Such knowledge is essential in considering the possible contributions of plausible rival hypotheses to the study's observed outcomes. While this is well accepted for quasi-experimental studies, it is also true in experiments using randomized assignment to treatment. Too often, researchers make the mistake of trusting too heavily in random assignment to defeat the action of possible rival hypotheses. In the drawing of experimental conclusions, randomization—although one of the researcher's most powerful tools—cannot be expected to replace thorough understanding of the events and experiences of the experiment's various groups. For example, experimental and control subjects may all be receiving treatment from similar programs outside the experimental environment; thus, group differences that would otherwise be created by the experimental treatment are obscured. A measurement-related example of this point would concern a flu virus that sweeps through a school population, setting back data collection for some or all participating students by, say, two weeks—enough time for some immediate treatment effects to partially dissipate. Social science practice sometimes operates as if quantitative methodologies make such knowing unnecessary, but this position is a serious error (Campbell, 1978).

6. *Funding of cross-validational research as part of program dissemination.* Once a funded research project develops a health program and finds it to be effective through a series of controlled field trials, that program ideally should be disseminated to a wide audience of potential program adopters, be they schools, clinics, community organizations, or other appropriate units. As described earlier, this is one critical stage in which attention to evaluation typically breaks down, yet it is during dissemination and diffusion that much can be learned about a program's ultimate effectiveness and value. Details of implementation, audience, and situational context will undoubtedly vary widely across program sites, and this natural variation offers an unparalleled opportunity to study the robustness of a program and the factors that mediate its effectiveness.

To encourage evaluation activity during the diffusion process, we recommend that funders of health research (such as government agencies and foundations) plan early to offer funding for some relevant form of evaluation in the adoption sites, should a program reach the dissemination stage. This evaluation activity should be conducted uniformly in terms of measurement instruments (or items), testing modalities, time-frames, and so on. In this way, a process of cross-validation can be established that will permit a much richer understanding of the health program's strengths and weaknesses and will inform practitioners' decisions about whether to implement the program in a particular setting.

7. *The use of meta-analysis.* As the number of formal evaluations of health promotion programs grows, the meta-analytical approach becomes increasingly important as a tool for interpreting the accumulating body of knowledge. In recent years, there have been several meta-analyses of smoking, alcohol and drug abuse prevention programs (Rundall and Bruvold, 1988; Tobler, 1986). This approach typically requires detailed experimental information, sometimes including raw data, to produce maximum validity. In the interest of accountability, scientific cross-validation, and the optimal utilization of research, projects should make their data records available for these analyses. This is particularly true for government-funded projects. A project's funding agency is one possible resource for archiving its data tapes. Insofar as projects often under-analyze the data they collect, these data records could also be used for secondary analyses, increasing the utility of the research effort.

8. *Encouragement of self-criticism and disclosure.* As described earlier, governmental priorities, media attention, and erratic funding, as well as other factors associated with prevention efforts in drug abuse and other health areas, create substantial pressures on social scientists to produce reports of effective programs and unambiguous findings. Thus, researchers may be tempted to obscure problems with experimental design, treatment implementation, or other elements of an intervention's field trials. Obviously, these temptations must be discouraged, although it would be naive to suggest that they can be completely removed.

Nevertheless, there are several actions that agencies can take to encourage an ethic of self-criticism and open discussion of research problems. First, agencies can make it clear to their grantees, through their original requests for proposals and other written communications, that they expect research difficulties to be encountered, openly dealt with, and documented. Second, they can require that research reports include a section that details specific difficulties that were experienced and the resolutions attempted, as well as recommendations for adjusting the original experimental design, were the study to be reattempted. Third, they can create a policy allowing all professional research staff members on a project team to have access to project data for reanalysis and potential publication (Campbell, 1984); such a policy, clearly diverging from the current norm of unified project reports, could serve to create a self-monitoring atmosphere within each team. Fourth, funding agencies can arrange forums specifically for the examination of such common (and uncommon) research problems as population coverage, treatment attrition, demand characteristics on measurement instruments, and so on.

The National Cancer Institute's Smoking, Tobacco, and Cancer Program (within its Division of Cancer Prevention and Control) in recent years has instituted a practice that facilitates the sharing of problems, solutions, and assorted ideas among its grantee projects. It brings its funded investigators together on an annual basis to report to and consult with one another on their research. This approach can contribute strongly to a shared consideration of theoretical and methodological issues, in a context that offers more timeliness and practicality than such other avenues as professional conferences and publication in journals. (Nevertheless, this approach can create some tendency toward methodological identity between projects, which has costs as well as benefits.)

9. Publication of research proposals and critiques. Substantial creativity and effort are expended in the process of preparing and reviewing proposals. There is no a priori reason (given appropriate timeframes) why the audience for this important work needs to be limited to the individuals directly involved in the granting decisions. In fact, such limitation can lead to an undesirable insulation of ideas in that only those researchers invited to serve as reviewers gain exposure to the range of projects being proposed and to the institutions' responses. This breadth of perspective would seem to give reviewers a natural advantage in later proposal cycles. Furthermore, proposals judged worthy, but for which funds are unavailable, are given no avenue to advance thinking in the field as a whole.

Therefore, we recommend that a journal, monograph series, or other form of publication be introduced for intervention researchers. This publication would include research proposals (or sections thereof) and accompanying critiques, as well as articles related to issues of experimental design, methodology, budget management, researcher-sponsor relationships, and a host of other topics of importance to the research community. For scientists actively involved in the proposal process, such a forum devoted to the *planning* of intervention research would undoubtedly be a valuable adjunct to the established focus on retrospective reporting of research efforts.

10. Long-term follow-up of intervention efforts. As we have discussed, stakeholders in the legislative and public sectors have very limited tolerance for long evaluation studies that may postpone programmatic action by several years. In addition, the substantial methodological problems associated with long-term follow-up are well documented in the research literature (for example, see Biglan and others, 1987; Campbell, 1988; Cook, 1985). Nevertheless, researchers are in strong agreement that long-term follow-up is essential to determining whether a program has contributed to a lasting change in individual behavior, in organizational functioning, or in some other variable of interest. Sponsoring agencies need to build this priority into their funded projects. Given the aforementioned realities, they should also encourage researchers to develop and use theoretical models that incorporate proximal mediators of these long-term outcomes.

An investigation of the problems associated with long-term follow-up—and strategies for their resolution—would be highly beneficial to researchers working across a range of health promotion areas. One component of such an investigation could involve experimental manipulation—looking at, say, the effectiveness of a variety of mail-contact strategies for long-term maintenance of subjects' addresses and consent. Another component, equally important, could be a compilation of interviews with experienced research teams regarding their perceptions of the major threats to experimental validity and how these can be addressed, either logistically or (if necessary) statistically. In addition, this investigation could explore what kinds of institutional arrangements are best suited to carrying out repeated follow-ups most efficiently.

Conclusion

This chapter has addressed current health promotion research and program development from the perspective of the sociology of science. Social scientists in this field operate under difficult conditions, including strong public pressures and limited coordination of research. We have proposed several recommendations related to the organization and focus of research efforts. We believe that further development of these themes can benefit the coordination of applied social science researchers working in these areas, with benefits also for the quality of research and intervention programming.

References

Bales, J. "Drug Funding: Now You See It . . ." *APA Monitor,* February 1987, pp. 15–16.

Best, J. A., Thomson, S. J., Santi, S. M., Smith, E. A., and Brown, K. S. "Preventing Cigarette Smoking Among School Children." *Annual Review of Public Health,* 1988, *9,* 161–201.

Biglan, A., Severson, H., Ary, D., Faller, C., Gallison, C., Thompson, R., Glasgow, R., and Lichtenstein, E. "Do Smoking Prevention Programs Really Work? Attrition and the Internal and External Validity of an Evaluation of a Refusal Skills Training Program." *Journal of Behavioral Medicine,* 1987, *10* (2), 159–171.

Campbell, D. T. "Qualitative Knowing in Action Research." In M. Brenner, P. Marsh, and M. Brenner (eds.), *The Social Contexts of Method.* London: Croom Helm, 1978.

Campbell, D. T. "Can We Be Scientific in Applied Social Science?" In R. F. Conner, D. G. Altman, and C. Jackson (eds.), *Evaluation Studies Review Annual.* Vol. 9. Newbury Park, Calif.: Sage, 1984.

Campbell, D. T. "Relabeling Internal and External Validity for Applied Social Scientists." In W.M.K. Trochim (ed.), *Advances in Quasi-Experimental Design and Analysis.* New Directions for Program Evaluation, no. 31. San Francisco: Jossey-Bass, 1986a.

Campbell, D. T. "Science's Social System of Validity-Enhancing Collective Belief Change and the Problems of the Social Sciences." In D. W. Fiske and R. A. Shweder (eds.), *Metatheory in Social Science: Pluralisms and Subjectivities.* Chicago: University of Chicago Press, 1986b.

Campbell, D. T. "Guidelines for Monitoring the Scientific Competence of Preventive Intervention Research Centers: An Exercise in the Sociology of Scientific Validity." *Knowledge: Creation, Diffusion, Utilization,* 1987, *8* (3), 389–430.

Campbell, D. T. (E. S. Overman, ed.) *Methodology and Epistemology for Social Sciences: Selected Papers.* Chicago: University of Chicago Press, 1988.

Cook, T. D. "Priorities in Research in Smoking Prevention." In C. S. Bell and R. Battjes (eds.), *Prevention Research: Deterring Drug Abuse Among Children and Adolescents.* NIDA Research Monograph, no. 63. Rockville, Md.: National Institute on Drug Abuse, 1985.

Cook, T. D., and Campbell, D. T. *Quasi-Experimentation: Design and Analysis Issues for Field Settings.* Skokie, Ill.: Rand McNally, 1979.

⚹ Evans, R. I. "Health Promotion—Science or Ideology?" *Health Psychology,* 1988, *7* (3), 203–219.

Goodstadt, M. S. "Prevention Strategies for Drug Abuse." *Issues in Science and Technology,* 1987, *4* (2), 28–35.

Janicki, T., and Braverman, M. T. "The Development and Evaluation of School Smoking Prevention Programs." In W. B. Ward (ed.), *Advances in Health Education and Promotion.* Vol. 1-B. Greenwich, Conn.: JAI Press, 1986.

Klitzner, M. D. "An Assessment of the Research on School-Based Prevention Programs." In U.S. Department of Education, *Report to Congress and the White House on the Nature and Effectiveness of Federal, State, and Local Drug Prevention/Education Programs.* Washington, D.C.: U.S. Department of Education, 1987.

McCaul, K. D., and Glasgow, R. E. "Preventing Adolescent Smoking: What Have We Learned About Treatment Construct Validity?" *Health Psychology,* 1985, *4,* 361–387.

Morrison, D. R., and Sivilli, J. "A Summary of Federal Drug Abuse Education and Prevention Programs for Youth." In U.S. Department of Education, *Report to Congress and the White House on the Nature and Effectiveness of Federal, State, and Local Drug Prevention/Education Programs.* Washington, D.C.: U.S. Department of Education, 1987.

Moskowitz, J. M. "The Primary Prevention of Alcohol Problems: A Critical Review of the Research Literature." *Journal of Studies on Alcohol,* 1989, *50,* 54–88.

Pollin, W. "Drug Abuse, U.S.A.: How Serious? How Soluble?" *Issues in Science and Technology,* 1987, *4* (2), 20–27.

Rundall, T. G., and Bruvold, W. H. "A Meta-Analysis of School-Based Smoking and Alcohol Use Prevention Programs." *Health Education Quarterly,* 1988, *15* (3), 317–334.

Tobler, N. "Meta-Analysis of 143 Adolescent Drug Prevention Programs: Quantitative Outcome Results of Program Participants Compared to a Control or Comparison Group." *Journal of Drug Issues,* 1986, *16,* 537–567.

U.S. Congress, House of Representatives. *Select Committee on Narcotics Abuse and Control, Hearings May 20–21, 1986.* Washington, D.C.: U.S. Government Printing Office, 1987.

U.S. Department of Education. *What Works: Schools Without Drugs.* Washington, D.C.: U.S. Department of Education, 1986.

U.S. Department of Education. *Report to Congress and the White House on the*

18

Nature and Effectiveness of Federal, State, and Local Drug Prevention/Education Programs. Washington, D.C.: U.S. Department of Education, 1987.

U.S. Department of Health and Human Services. *The 1990 Health Objectives for the Nation: A Midcourse Review.* Washington, D.C.: U.S. Government Printing Office, 1986.

U.S. General Accounting Office. "Implementation of the Drug-Free Schools and Communities Act." Briefing document 104590. Unpublished report, U.S. General Accounting Office, 1987.

Wallack, L., and Corbett, K. "Alcohol, Tobacco, and Marijuana Use Among Youth: An Overview of Epidemiological, Program, and Policy Trends." *Health Education Quarterly,* 1987, *14* (2), 223–249.

Marc T. Braverman is educational research and evaluation specialist for the University of California Cooperative Extension/4-H and a faculty member in human development at the University of California, Davis.

Donald T. Campbell is university professor of social relations, psychology, and education at Lehigh University. He is a member of the National Academy of Sciences and past president of the American Psychological Association. He is also a former recipient of the Myrdal Prize in Science of the Evaluation Research Society.

Community health intervention methods, objectives, and contexts are linked to evaluation issues, and some options for addressing these issues are suggested.

Evaluating Community-Level Health Promotion and Disease Prevention Interventions

Christine Jackson, David G. Altman, Beth Howard-Pitney, John W. Farquhar

In the United States and elsewhere, communities are demonstrating increased political and economic support for programs that promote health and prevent disease. Contributing to this trend is the increased recognition that many of the leading causes of disability and premature death are in fact preventable and that the surrounding physical and social environment—that is, the community itself—influences health status. There has also been considerable growth in public concern about lifestyle-related health problems, including AIDS, elevated cholesterol, and tobacco smoke, resulting in increased demand at the local level for preventive interventions. With traditional health care systems lacking the technical and financial resources to respond to this demand, a diverse mix of public health, political, educational, industrial, commercial, civic, and other groups are attempting to meet the community need for health promotion and disease prevention.

Marc T. Braverman (ed.). *Evaluating Health Promotion Programs.*
New Directions for Program Evaluation, no. 43. San Francisco: Jossey-Bass, Fall 1989.

Among the earliest efforts by communities in the United States to implement health promotion and disease prevention programs were the federally funded demonstration trials for reducing cardiovascular disease risk (Blackburn, 1983; Farquhar, Fortmann, Wood, and Haskell, 1983). During the nearly twenty pioneering years that have elapsed since the initiation of these trials, considerable progress has occurred in developing effective interventions and strategies for communities to implement them. One of the lessons learned during this period is that the complex etiology of preventable outcomes, such as cardiovascular disease or alcohol misuse, necessitates a correspondingly complex intervention plan and evaluation design. This evolution of complex preventive community interventions has tested the limits of all aspects of evaluation research. Evaluators face significant challenges in developing sampling, measurement, design, and implementation strategies that can survive the complexity of community interventions with enough conceptual and methodological integrity to justify the effort. This chapter describes some of these challenges and options for meeting them.

A theme we will raise at the close of the chapter is that the options for conducting scientifically sound evaluations of community-level interventions are currently quite limited. Our perspective is that there is a need for evaluators who understand and accept the realities of community-level intervention, who are willing to design evaluations that do not ignore these realities, and who therefore have the potential to devise methods that improve the scientific soundness of community evaluation methods.

Community Health Interventions

All health promotion and disease prevention interventions are not alike, and which evaluation issues are relevant depends on the characteristics of the intervention. We therefore begin our discussion of evaluation issues with a broad description of what we mean by the term *community health intervention.*

Our focus is on interventions that have primary prevention objectives and not, for example, treatment or health service utilization objectives. Because of their preventive orientation, the principal beneficiaries of these interventions are the healthy members of a community. These interventions aim to reduce the incidence rate within the community of diseases and disabilities that have modifiable causal conditions. They conceptualize solutions to health problems as these are related to an array of biological, psychological, cultural, social, and regulatory factors, and they attempt to reach all members of the target population via a comprehensive set of integrated program elements. A community intervention intended, for example, to reduce the rate of elevated blood cholesterol may attempt to change knowledge and beliefs regarding dietary fat and cholesterol, food selection and preparation, physicians' screening and treatment practices, school nutrition curricula, the foods available in markets, nutrition policies in worksite cafeterias and restaurants, and food-labeling laws. As exemplified here, implementation of community interventions typically occurs across multiple settings, using multiple change strategies, to achieve broad and repeated exposure to a set of complementary and interdependent activities. Finally, community health interventions often have an underlying philosophy of self-determination, as evidenced by a high degree of local control over the purpose and scope of the intervention and, often, over the evaluation.

Evaluation Issues

The evaluation issues we have identified can be attributed to one of three facets of community health intervention: the complexity of the intervention methods, the health promotion and disease prevention objectives, and the community context in which these interventions occur. What follows is a discussion of what we believe to be among the most challenging evaluation issues associated with each of these facets of community health intervention.

Complex Intervention Methods. Among the most salient characteristics of community interventions is the complexity of their treatment processes. This complexity is intentional and is intended to achieve the synergistic effects that are assumed to result when mutually reinforcing activities occur across multiple levels and settings in a community. This complexity is also the root cause of several significant design and measurement issues.

Conceptualizing the Unit of Intervention. One implication of the complexity of community interventions is that evaluators have some latitude in conceptualizing the unit of intervention (that is, the unit within which the effects of the intervention are expected to occur). To understand this issue, consider the following set of activities, all of which could be simultaneously implemented in a community to reduce the rate of cigarette smoking: One activity provides individual smokers with self-help cessation materials; another institutes a peer-resistance program in school curricula; another trains physicians to facilitate patients' cessation efforts; another enables restaurants, markets, hospitals, and worksites to establish nonsmoking ordinances; another uses mass media to increase support within the community for a state tobacco-tax initiative. Is this one smoking intervention or several? If it is one intervention, at what level is it occurring (what is the unit of intervention), and how can its overall effects be tested?

The answers to these conceptual questions set an important cornerstone in the development of the evaluation plan. As noted by Cook (1985), assumptions regarding the nature of the intervention (for example, its diffusibility and potential to affect such community-level factors as norms), along with other considerations (for example, sample size and reliability of measures), guide decisions regarding the appropriate unit of analysis for the evaluation. If one assumes that the unit being treated by or exposed to an intervention is the whole community, then the conceptually appropriate unit of analysis for the test of the effects of that intervention would be the community.

While many who implement and evaluate community interventions agree with the concept of the community as the optimal unit of investigation, the costs of recruiting and studying a sufficiently large sample of communities are generally prohibitive. Thus, in practice, evaluations of community interventions generally treat smaller units (say, individuals or organizations) as the units of analysis. One concern regarding use of units of analysis smaller than the unit of intervention is that the resultant increase in degrees of freedom may reduce the estimates of the standard errors and make statistically significant results more likely (Cook, 1985). A second concern that arises when one relies on data from units other than communities is that communities are unique in ways that may confound the effect of a health promotion intervention. This occurs largely because the presence of individuals and organizations within a community is not random but instead is determined by a composite of personal, social, economic, and environmental considerations. Communities therefore vary in population size and demography, in economic base, in exposure to mass media, in presence of hospitals, health departments, universities, and other institutions, and in other factors with the potential to bias the effect of an intervention. It is difficult to obtain valid assessments of intervention effects when the influence of such community-level variables is not taken into account.

There are design options that, to varying degrees, address these concerns and stay within the resource limitations of most evaluations. Evaluators may obtain data from fewer but well-matched communities and establish the comparability of the communities by intensive assessment of the potential sources of community-level bias. A modification of this approach is, again, to establish the homogeneity of the communities but to increase power by collecting relatively fewer data from a greater number of communities. When it is not possible to have comparison communities, evaluators may have to rely solely on prepost comparisons of within-treatment community data to estimate intervention effects. Such evaluations should strive to take full advantage of designs (for example, interrupted time series or regression discontinuity; Cook and Campbell, 1979) that can be applied within a treatment community and still yield a true indication of treatment effects. For these designs to be viable, planning for the evaluation and the program needs to occur simultaneously and well in advance of program implementation.

Another within-community option, which may be feasible when the evaluator can influence program implementation, is to apply block designs to establish no-treatment samples within a single community. For example, one may delay intervention in some census tracts, neighborhoods, or other community segments that (ideally) are matched and randomly assigned to a delayed-treatment control. Considerable opportunity exists to improve the integrity of this option by developing alternative within-community sampling units. It may be possible to apply social area analysis (Struening, 1983) to identify geographically distinct areas within a community that are conceptually meaningful in terms of how subpopulations (including persons and settings) interact with a health promotion intervention; that is, it may be possible to define a unit larger than individuals or organizations, but smaller than entire communities, whose responses to a community-level intervention are independent and comparable.

These are just some of the possible modifications to the optimal but generally unattainable design that compares a large sample of homogeneous, randomly assigned treated and untreated communities. Despite its generally low feasibility, this design serves as an important conceptual reference point against which the strengths and weaknesses of these and other design options can be assessed. In particular, it serves to underscore the need to evaluate sources of community-level bias that may influence the treatment effect and to avoid attributing to communities results based on individual-level or group-level data.

Not all who implement a community health intervention will conceptualize it as a single independent variable operating at the community level; that is, a comprehensive intervention may be implemented but conceptualized as several independently evaluable programs. This situation frequently occurs because program planners often maintain two goals: They want to maximize the probability that the intervention will make a difference, and therefore they implement a comprehensive intervention; and they are keenly interested in learning which components of the intervention did or did not contribute to the overall intervention effects. The problem is that these goals are not entirely compatible. The greater the success in implementing a comprehensive, interactive set of intervention activities, the more difficult it becomes to design evaluations that provide valid assessments of the independent contribution of a single intervention activity. Trying to evaluate program-specific effects within the context of several other intentionally interactive programs increases the potential for confounded data. Thus, while it is feasible and desirable within the framework of a comprehensive intervention to collect thorough process data on specific intervention components, program-specific outcome evaluations are best conducted in settings without ongoing comprehensive interventions.

Working Across Disciplines. The complexity of community intervention methods raises other evaluation issues. One issue is that substantive knowledge from many disciplines is required to conduct evaluations of comprehensive programs. Consider the cholesterol and smoking interventions described earlier, which may produce change in biological, psychological, behavioral, sociocultural, regulatory, and environmental variables. Establishing the measurement criteria and developing the measurement tools to evaluate these effects would require knowledge from such disciplines as social psychology, communications, medicine, and nutrition, as well as knowledge of research design, sampling methods, and data analysis. Such evaluations also require familiarity with the structure and dynamics of community systems, such as the educational, commercial, industrial, and political systems. Community health interventions challenge evaluators either to have a broad base of knowledge or to recruit a multidisciplinary team of consultants or colleagues. They also require outside evaluators who can learn enough about the composition of a community to identify feasible mechanisms for data collection and to estimate the stability of community factors that, if changed, could modify intervention effects.

Monitoring Diffused Intervention Processes. Community health interventions frequently utilize indirect or diffused methods of program implementation; that is, the primary targets of the intervention may not be the general population but the providers, gatekeepers, and opinion leaders in the community. An intervention may target physicians (who then reach patients), teachers (who then reach students), business and union leaders (who then reach employees), and owners of such commercial establishments as restaurants and markets (who then reach customers). Having reached the primary target groups, the intervention may encourage the members of these groups to carry out direct intervention among their constituencies (as when physicians counsel patients to quit smoking, or when worksites sponsor fitness programs for employees). Alternatively, the intervention may have as secondary targets, not individuals, but environmental variables under the control of the primary target group (for example, worksite smoking policies or food preparation practices in restaurants).

Diffused methods of intervention generate some evaluation demands that are fairly straightforward but none the less challenging. To document program implementation and monitor exposure to the intervention, evaluators need to spend considerable time modeling the persons, places, and change objectives that comprise each target sequence. One sequence could be training teachers to train student peer-group leaders to lead peer groups through a program on resisting pressures to smoke. Much theoretical and logistical information is needed to plan and manage the process monitoring of several such sequences that have different timelines and involve different population subgroups and community systems.

Utilizing Multiple Data Collection Methods. To capture the effects of a comprehensive intervention, evaluators generally must utilize several data collection methods. The Stanford Five-City Project (Farquhar and others, 1985), for example, utilized physiological measures, questionnaires, face-to-face interviews, telephone surveys, observational study, and review of archival data (hospital records) as evaluation tools. When multiple data collection instruments are used, evaluators should develop data collection systems that allow comparison of data across data sets so that convergent (or divergent) evidence for an effect can be established. One may expect, for example, to find convergence between organizational-level data on sponsorship of cholesterol screenings and individual-level data on the perceived availability and rate of utilization of cholesterol screenings. This type of sender-receiver comparison is possible when items of similar content are included in instruments to be used for different response groups and/or at different levels of the community. This approach allows for cross-checking of results and so increases one's confidence in the interpretation of the results.

Measuring Environmental Variables. Evaluation of community interventions will probably require measurement of such environmental variables as worksite health promotion activities, school curricula, city smoking ordinances, and community exercise facilities. There is little previous work to draw on in trying to develop the sampling frames and data collection methods for most environmental variables; for example, few sources identify all of the worksites in a community and stratify them by type of business or number of employees. The available data are also likely to be outdated or otherwise incomplete (for example, Chamber of Commerce listings) or nearly complete but very expensive to obtain (for example, Dun & Bradstreet data tapes). Having established an organizational-level sample, one then needs to devise strategies for extracting data from the organizations. A problem we have faced consistently in this regard is that only the rare organization has members who are knowledgeable about the complete set of activities that occur in the organization. We have found that school district supervisors or school principals generally are unable to report on teaching activity for a specific health topic, and a single teacher can usually report only on his or her own teaching activity. Similarly, it is unusual to find any one person at a worksite, hospital, health department, or city government who can provide accurate or detailed information on the provision or utilization of health promotion resources. Few organizations record these data, and those that do are unlikely to record information pertinent to the evaluation.

There is a need to improve our capacity to measure organizational-level and community-level variables. It may be possible to develop new methods (or apply existing methods from other fields) that sample several individuals and/or archives to generate a collective estimate of organizational activity. Another promising approach would be to develop software programs that facilitate the tracking of health promotion activities by community organizations or groups. A third approach, already receiving considerable attention, is developing social indicators of community health promotion activity (Andrews, in press; Flora, Jackson, and Maccoby, in press; Rundall, 1988). Briefly, the object of this research is to assess community-level variables, such as restaurant sales of heart-healthy meals or expenditures in a community for AIDS education, which may be expected to change as a result of an intervention. Indicator variables often do not provide complete or direct assessment of the criterion variable but instead provide reliable, valid indications of fluctuation in that variable. Restaurant sales of healthy meals, for example, would not be a measure of dietary fat consumption but could provide an indication of changes in dietary fat consumption. Collection of indicator data often involves archival and unobtrusive data collection methods, which can be relatively inexpensive. Indicator variables may therefore increase the feasibility of conducting longitudinal studies of program effects, as well as providing a means to measure community response to an intervention.

Health Promotion and Disease Prevention Objectives. A second facet of community health interventions that gives rise to evaluation issues is their health promotion and disease prevention objectives. Interventions with these objectives are often characterized by voluntary participation in intervention activities, limited denial of access to the intervention, and gradual, long-term change processes. These characteristics have important implications for evaluation.

Voluntary Intervention. Interventions intended to prevent the occurrence of a negative health outcome necessarily target persons who have not yet experienced any of the harmful or unpleasant effects associated with the health threat. Thus, compared to individuals with a diagnosed illness or known family history of a hereditary disease, the majority of potential beneficiaries of preventive interventions have more choice and face less urgency about involvement in health promotion and disease prevention activities. Similarly, most community organizations, such as worksites, schools, or civic groups voluntarily engage in health promotion activities.

From an evaluation perspective, there is a significant cost associated with the voluntary aspect of prevention activities. When each person, group, and organization in the community is free to participate in whichever combination of intervention activities is of interest, it is not possible to standardize exposure to the intervention. From the target population's perspective, a community health intervention is not one intervention but is as many interventions as there are permutations of the programmatic activities that occur.

One way to compensate for this extreme form of selection bias is to use statistical controls—that is, to collect sufficient data to utilize multivariate analyses that control for selection effects. Given this strategy, process evaluation must do more than determine whether the program was implemented as planned. It must also measure exposure to the intervention activities for each unit of intervention (for example, person, household, or school) and participant characteristics that may confound treatment effects, including sociodemographics and such likely covariates of program participation as perceived self-efficacy, group norms, baseline levels of school health curricula, and size of worksite. Such process evaluation data are important outcomes in their own right and are potentially critical sources of covariates for explaining summative evaluation measures. The limiting factors of this approach are high costs, the strong likelihood of unknowingly excluding important covariates, and decreased interpretability of data included in the multivariate analyses. These limitations should be compared to the conceptual and financial costs of establishing no-treatment controls. Such controls, if well matched, should allow a design in which the effects of selection variables on program involvement and impact are balanced. Of course, the combined use of intensive process evaluation and no-treatment controls is optimal.

Ethical Limits to Establishing Controls. Community health interventions that target chronic disease risk factors generally are not initiated until sufficient epidemiological and biomedical data are available to identify the risk factors and to link changes in risk factors with changes in the probability of the disease. Once disease prevention recommendations are made at the national level, as has been done for cancer and cardiovascular disease risk factors (although not without controversy—see Becker, 1987), denial of access to risk-reduction interventions for research purposes becomes difficult to justify on ethical grounds. While community members generally are supportive of evaluation research, they may be unwilling to deny or delay program access to segments of the community to accommodate the research agenda. Because of this ethical concern and other client concerns (for example, public relations), a random no-treatment control group from within an intervention community is a rare component of evaluations of community health interventions. Although establishing outside controls is one alternative, it is an option that does not entirely satisfy the ethical concern regarding access to preventive intervention, and it probably will require a firm commitment to provide the same intervention upon completion of the evaluation. Thus, while resource-limitation issues push the evaluator toward establishing control groups within the intervention community, the ethics of denying prevention programs may cause the evaluator to turn to outside communities for control groups or to evaluate without control groups.

Long-Term Intervention Objectives. Programs that strive to reduce the incidence of an unhealthful event often have a substantial time lag between the start of intervention and any measurable effect on program goals. One would expect, for example, at least fifteen years to pass before one could measure the effects of a prevention program for heart disease on morbidity and mortality rates. A shorter but nevertheless substantial period separates changes in sexual practices and the incidence of AIDS. This issue further underscores the need for evaluators to understand well the pathogenesis and epidemiology of the target disease or health problem. It also underscores the need for accurate modeling of the causal paths that link antecedent conditions to the disease or health problem. This knowledge is needed to identify the critical interim variables and their associated points in time along the etiological process, and to establish a series of measures of program effects that coincide with those points. Given limited resources, those planning the evaluation need to reconcile the trade-off between obtaining comprehensive information at a few points and obtaining considerably less information at multiple points.

Community as Stakeholder. The third facet of community health interventions that gives rise to evaluation issues is that entire communities, often represented by coalitions of community organizations, may maintain a stake in both the intervention and its evaluation. The members of such a stakeholder group typically have diverse interests and experience in health intervention and evaluation research, as well as a long history of interacting on other community projects. This section discusses some steps that evaluators can take to work more effectively with a heterogeneous, highly interactive group of community stakeholders.

Gain Consensus on the Objectives of the Evaluation. Evaluators and stakeholders alike must reach early agreement on the objectives of the evaluation; that is, they must agree on the questions the evaluation will answer. Although this is an elementary step in evaluation methodology, it is a step easily compromised in community-level evaluations. Evaluators and stakeholders frequently agree on generalities about the purpose of an evaluation but fail to reach consensus on the specific questions an evaluation will address. This can occur because a heterogeneous group of stakeholders may identify several (sometimes competing) evaluation objectives, and they may disagree on which objectives should take precedence. Stakeholders may find it difficult, for example, to set priorities for conducting an intensive evaluation of subgroups within the community versus conducting a less informative evaluation of the entire community. Similarly, stakeholders may disagree on the relative importance of process evaluation data versus outcome evaluation data, or short-term versus long-term outcome data. Moreover, it is likely that the composition of the stakeholder group will change during the course of the evaluation, introducing new expectations regarding evaluation objectives.

Gaining consensus among stakeholders is in fact only the first part of a long process; the true challenge for evaluators is to maintain consensus and commitment once evaluation objectives are specified. Among the factors contributing to erosion of support for evaluation objectives is that stakeholders often underestimate the time and effort needed to meet an objective, and their support may wane as the true costs of conducting the evaluation become apparent. Also undermining support for a given objective is the conflict that stakeholders may experience between their commitment to both the intervention and the evaluation. When evaluation objectives can be achieved only at some cost to the intervention objectives, stakeholders may begin to question the utility of the evaluation and experience some confusion about whether and how to meet both sets of objectives.

A key contributor to the problem of consensus development among stakeholders is that stakeholders generally are not experts in evaluation. They do not have the information necessary to frame evaluation questions or anticipate the steps and compromises required to answer these questions. Even though stakeholders may lack the knowledge to make informed evaluation decisions, they are likely to have substantial input in the decision-making process. The potential for conflict is apparent. Equally apparent is that program evaluators who want to work collaboratively with stakeholders need to dedicate some time to providing them with sufficient information to enable them to contribute to evaluation planning and sustain a commitment to the evaluation process. Added benefits of this effort are that the accumulation of evaluation knowledge by stakeholders improves their capacity to be advocates for the evaluation, to be responsible for components of the evaluation, and to utilize the evaluation data.

Develop a Systems Perspective on the Community. An easily overlooked step in working with communities is developing a general understanding of what a community is and a specific understanding of the persons, places, and activities that comprise the community involved in the evaluation. Community-level evaluators need to understand both the community as a system and the dynamics of introducing a large-scale intervention into that system. Briefly, they need to know the patterns of interactions, or networks of persons and organizations, within the community. They need to know the norms and rules that govern these interactions, as well as the community's established methods for allocation of its relatively stable quantity of resources. Most important, evaluators should recognize that the introduction of a comprehensive health intervention is a disturbance of the community system since it seeks to change the status quo, reallocate resources, and alter existing norms.

Evaluators who develop a systems perspective on communities are better prepared to work with stakeholders as collaborators and decision makers in the evaluation. Depending on his or her role within the community system, a stakeholder will work to structure the evaluation that best accommodates (or least threatens) the needs of his or her organization or constituency. Stakeholders, for example, can assist an evaluation by providing knowledge of and access to critical data, or they can hinder an evaluation by rejecting the use of random assignment or failing to support specific data collection efforts. The support that stakeholders provide to an evaluation is influenced by their interests and accountabilities within the community system. An evaluator who knows the community can anticipate these interests and accountabilities and is generally better prepared to work collaboratively with stakeholders to plan an evaluation compatible with the larger community agenda.

Be Prepared for Uncontrollable Events. No matter how well informed the community stakeholders and how genuine the collaboration between stakeholders and evaluators, the dynamic nature of community systems can suddenly and dramatically alter the intervention and its evaluation. An intervention with overlapping objectives may be initiated by another group in the community. Control communities may initiate programs. A sudden local increase in the rate of politically "hot" health problems (AIDS, drug use, drinking and driving, adolescent pregnancy) may cause an equally sudden shift in intervention activity or evaluation funding. Teachers, for example, may be directed to devote all health education time to AIDS education, usurping time initially committed to nutrition education. There is little that evaluators and stakeholders can do to prevent these events. They can, however, be prepared for their occurrence and, when stakeholders agree it is appropriate, utilize the available evaluation data to dissuade others from disrupting the ongoing intervention and its evaluation.

Anticipate Utilization Needs. Community stakeholders often require simple answers to complex questions, which is to say that they need usable data from the evaluation. Thus, while the intervention program may be complex and the evaluation system correspondingly complex, interpretation and presentation of the data generally need to be straightforward to be useful in the community context. This is particularly true when data are to be used in the political arena as leverage for future program decisions. What is most useful in this situation is often a single statistic of a program's effects. In this regard, the cost-to-effect ratio is emerging as an increasingly important criterion for the comparable value of community health promotion interventions.

Conclusion

Our intent in this chapter has been to convey the nature of the conceptual and methodological issues faced by evaluators of comprehensive community health interventions. The issues we have raised are pertinent to the evaluation of most community interventions. We believe, however, that these issues are more pronounced in communitywide health interventions and, within this arena, test the limits of current evaluation concepts and methods. Another way of making this point is to consider communitywide health interventions in light of Lipsey's (1988) "continuum of causal complexity." This continuum is anchored at one end by unidimensional, undifferentiated treatments applied at single points in time and at the other end by multidimensional treatments with variable causal processes applied over long periods of time. As defined in this chapter, community health interventions represent the extreme, complex end of the continuum. Lipsey's thesis is that as treatment processes become more complex, evaluators' capacity to define constructs, to operationalize constructs into valid, reliable, sensitive measures, and to avoid error in drawing conclusions becomes correspondingly more limited. The added complexity of community interventions is therefore not simply a matter of making familiar evaluation issues a bit more problematic; it is a matter of going beyond the adequacy of current evaluation concepts and methods.

Evaluators can begin to address this general issue—first, by wider use of the options now available, such as measurement of community bias covariates and use of time-series and regression-discontinuity designs. Second, more effort should be devoted to developing new options, such as using social area analysis, developing social indicator variables, and instituting tracking systems to measure organizational-level change. Third, there is a need for more evaluators to accept and work within the realities of community intervention, rather than trying to apply evaluation methods that ignore these realities. The much-needed innovations in the evaluation of comprehensive community-level programs are most likely to come from those whose thinking is as complex as the programs under investigation.

References

✗ Andrews, F. M. "Developing Indicators of Health Promotion: Contributions of the Social Indicator Movement." In S. B. Kar (ed.), *Proceedings of the Symposium on Indicators of Health-Promotion Behaviors*. New York: Springer, in press.

✗ Becker, M. H. "The Cholesterol Saga: Whither Health Promotion?" *Annals of Internal Medicine*, 1987, *106* (4) 623–625.

Blackburn, H. "Research and Demonstration Projects in Community Cardiovascular Disease Prevention." *Journal of Public Health Policy*, 1983, *4* (4), 398–421.

Cook, T. D. "Priorities in Research in Smoking Prevention." In C. S. Bell and R. Battjes (eds.), *Prevention Research: Deterring Drug Abuse Among Children and Adolescents*. NIDA Research Monograph, no. 63. Rockville, Md.: National Institute on Drug Abuse, 1985.

32

Cook, T. D., and Campbell, D. T. *Quasi-Experimentation: Design and Analysis Issues for Field Settings.* Skokie, Ill.: Rand McNally, 1979.

Farquhar, J. W., Fortmann, S. P., Maccoby, N., Haskell, W. L., Williams, P. T., Flora, J. A., Taylor, C. B., Brown, B. W., Solomon, D. S., and Hulley, S. B. "The Stanford Five-City Project: Design and Methods." *American Journal of Epidemiology*, 1985, *122* (2), 323–333.

Farquhar, J. W., Fortmann, S. P., Wood, P. D., and Haskell, W. L. "Community Studies of Cardiovascular Disease Prevention." In N. M. Kaplan and J. Stamler (eds.), *Prevention of Coronary Heart Disease.* Philadelphia: Saunders, 1983.

Flora, J. A., Jackson, C., and Maccoby, N. "Indicators of Societal Action to Promote Physical Health." In S. B. Kar (ed.), *Proceedings of the Symposium on Indicators of Health-Promotion Behaviors.* New York: Springer, in press.

Lipsey, M. W. "Practice and Malpractice in Evaluation Research." *Evaluation Practice*, 1988, *9* (4), 5–24.

Rundall, T. G. "Community Health Assessment: Measuring the Impact of Health Promotion." In Western Consortium for Public Health (ed.), *Health Promotion in California: A Compendium of Papers from California Health Promotion Consensus Project.* Berkeley, Calif.: Western Consortium for Public Health, 1988.

Struening, E. L. "Social Area Analysis as a Method of Evaluation." In E. L. Struening and M. B. Brewer (eds.), *Handbook of Evaluation Research.* Newbury Park, Calif.: Sage, 1983.

Christine Jackson is associate director of education for the Stanford Five-City Project. Her research interests include the analysis of social norms for health and the development of home-based health interventions.

David G. Altman is associate director of the Health Promotion Resource Center. His research focuses on tobacco policy, community health promotion, and program evaluation.

Beth Howard-Pitney is director of evaluation for the Health Promotion Resource Center, which provides consultation and technical assistance to communities engaged in community health interventions.

John W. Farquhar is director of the Stanford Center for Research in Disease Prevention. He has long been interested in researching community approaches to the prevention of heart disease.

*Health promoters need to change the ways in which they think
about program outcomes as programs progress through the
stages of research, development, and diffusion.*

Conceptualizing
Outcomes for Health
Promotion Programs

*J. Allan Best, K. Stephen Brown, Roy Cameron,
Edward A. Smith, Marjorie MacDonald*

As health promotion programs progress through the stages of research,
development, and diffusion, the nature of expected outcomes must
change. Three major problems are common in the conceptualizing of
outcomes:

1. Outcomes tend to focus on change in an individual's behavior.
   However, as program development and diffusion progress, *levels* of
   individual *and* system change must be considered.
2. Several factors act as *determinants* of intervention outcome, including content (the principles and activities prescribed by an intervention), participants (characteristics of individuals exposed to the
   program), providers (the characteristics and behavior of those delivering the program), and setting (the immediate and broader social
   and physical contexts in which interventions are delivered). We
   can intervene directly to modify any or all of these factors, and
   outcome measures can be developed to assess the short- and long-
   term effects of these interventions.

Marc T. Braverman (ed.). *Evaluating Health Promotion Programs.*
New Directions for Program Evaluation, no. 43. San Francisco: Jossey-Bass, Fall 1989.

3. Outcomes often are conceptualized as a state or event, rather than as a process that reflects *stages* of behavioral change. Research designs do not adequately address the time dimension inherent in health promotion processes.

The cube in Figure 1—showing levels, determinants, and stages—is adapted from Abrams and others (1986) and provided here as a tool for identifying the range of outcomes that could be measured in an evaluation. Health promotion programs increasingly aim to provide an integrated, multifactorial intervention that corresponds in complexity of intended effects to the complexity of determinants of health behavior and its change. Thus, outcomes are by design multiple, interrelated, and time-dependent.

The theses of this chapter are the following:

1. The definition and selection of outcomes must use a conceptual framework like the one in Figure 1.
2. The relative importance of the dimensions and cells changes through the research, development, and diffusion sequence.
3. It is useful to review constructs shown effective in predicting outcome at the individual level as a function of intervention content

Figure 1. Dimensions of Health Behavior Intervention

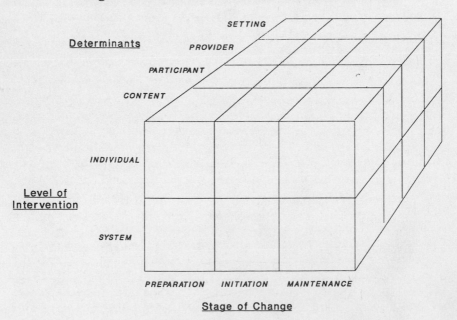

Note: Adapted from Abrams and others, 1986.

and participants to see if they can be adapted to provider and setting factors and to system levels of intervention. Social learning theory (Bandura, 1986) may be a useful tool in providing a parsimonious explanation of determinants at each level and of the relationships among them over time.

Our aim in this chapter is first to discuss this framework and the conceptual issues that flow from it and then to focus on implications for design and analysis. We draw heavily for examples on our smoking prevention and smoking cessation work, which has evolved through the research, development, and diffusion sequence over the last twenty years. However, we believe that the questions raised are generic to most health promotion intervention programs.

Stages of the Health Promotion Process

Health promotion intervention research moves from basic *research* that identifies determinants of health behavior and behavior change, to *development* of efficacious intervention methods, and finally to *diffusion* of the intervention. Several models have emerged in recent years to guide this process (Flay, 1986; Greenwald and Cullen, 1984; National Heart, Lung, and Blood Institute, 1983). These models address important design and measurement issues in research and development. However, program evaluation is particularly needed during diffusion, and none of these previously published models adequately addresses the diffusion stage. Diffusion itself can be viewed as involving four distinct steps, each with a different target audience and intervention objectives: dissemination (planned efforts to make policy makers and decision makers aware of health promotion innovations), adoption (interventions designed to encourage organizations to initiate a program), implementation (interventions for program providers designed to ensure that a program is implemented as intended), and maintenance (interventions targeting both decision makers and providers, to encourage retention and institutionalization of a program). Note that Figure 1 uses the stages of preparation, initiation, and maintenance, shown useful in describing processes of individual change, to describe what really is a very similar dimension. Diffusion is by its very nature a system-change intervention.

In sum, the type of research question, design, program target, intervention, and purpose or consumer of the research all change as research, development, and diffusion progress. There are major implications for choice of process and outcome measures, as illustrated throughout this chapter. In an ideal world, the progression would be well planned and carefully orchestrated. In practice, the literature reflects a breakdown at the transition between development and diffusion, as well as throughout the diffusion process.

In the first instance, the problem is at least twofold: (1) Relevant disciplines, methodologies, and funding sources all are changing simultaneously with the shift in focus from efficacy to effectiveness, and (2) there is a methodological choice to be made between extending clinical trial models to population/community systems research, on the one hand, and shifting to a program evaluation perspective, on the other. Clearly, we need to work toward the integration of these perspectives (Flay, 1986).

In the second instance, the problem arises from neglect. The researchers involved in developing and testing effective interventions rarely stay involved at the diffusion stage. As a consequence, outcomes often are not well conceptualized.

Implications of the Three-Dimensional Model

Levels of Intervention. Determinants of behavior and the behavioral change process should be conceived as different at the individual and systems levels. For example, consider smoking onset in youth at the individual level and at three levels of system. In doing so, note that Figure 1 simplifies the distinction between individual and system. In fact, many evaluations must come to terms with multiple levels of hierarchically nested systems.

At the individual level, biopsychosocial models describe influences on smoking onset (Best, Wainwright, Mills, and Kirkland, 1988). Biologically, individual factors include sensitivity to nicotine and the degree to which nicotine comes to serve important affect-regulation needs. A short-term program outcome could be whether a program teaches alternative strategies to cope with feelings and leads to an increase in the utilization of these coping behaviors in smoking situations. In the psychological and social realm, the influence of peers' perceived attitudes and behaviors is an important determinant (Chassin, Presson, and Sherman, 1984). An important program outcome could be changes in the perceived prevalence of same-age peer smoking.

At the family level, important factors may include family structure, cohesion, adaptability, and support (Best, in press). Some of these factors are amenable to intervention. For example, one outcome of a home-based curriculum for smoking prevention could be increased support or cohesion. A recent evaluation by Perry, Klepp, and Sillers (in press) found a significant short-term advantage for a home- versus school-based intervention, but there was decay of effects in subsequent years. Could increased support or cohesion be a necessary and sufficient mediating outcome for sustained effects?

At the institutional level, our data (Best and others, 1988) clearly show the importance of school environment, adjusting for other social influences (peers and family). We do not yet understand what determines these effects. Likely factors include norms (as reflected in smoking policies or in the priority placed on health education in the school), the degree of rule clarity and support in the school environment, and the modeling effects of older peer and staff smoking. Each of these school-environment determinants could be targeted for change and serve as an outcome measure.

Community is another systems level. The well-known heart health projects developed at Minnesota, Pawtucket, and Stanford intervene at this level (Blackburn and others, 1984; Farquhar and others, 1984; Lasater and others, 1984). The new U.S. National Cancer Institute Community Intervention Trial for Smoking Cessation (Pechacek, 1987) explicitly aims to produce and measure changes in community norms and operation. Perry, Luepker, Murray, and Hearn (in press) recently demonstrated that a school-based smoking prevention program was more effective in the context of a community heart health program.

What constructs are known to predict outcomes? These different levels of intervention and associated outcomes must be carefully linked, and causal processes must be explicitly stated. How can we usefully generalize constructs of established value at the individual level to system levels? Can the same constructs provide parsimonious, integrated frameworks for conceptualizing outcomes across levels as diffusion progresses?

The construct of social norms may have utility across the four levels illustrated in the smoking prevention example. The literature provides support for the value of Ajzen and Fishbein's (1980) perceived social norms for predicting behavior of individuals. We suggest that the construct is useful on systems levels as well: social norms as perceived by communities may powerfully affect behavior. For example, interventions designed to create the perception of a nonsmoking norm within a community may profoundly alter the behavior of smokers, as well as transactions between smokers and nonsmokers.

Another individual construct we find useful for generalizing to systems levels is capacity for change, which refers to the skills and resources necessary for behavioral change. At the individual level, this often is operationalized with constructs like self-efficacy and social support. At the population or community level, capacity for change may refer to the competence of program providers, the availability of physical resources, and the extent to which influential groups or individuals within the community modeled the desired behavior before intervention. Clearly, the concept needs refinement, but it illustrates an evolving conceptual framework that specifies key determinants and potential program outcomes on multiple levels.

These examples of individual constructs generalized to the systems level are only illustrative. Our intent is to argue the potential utility of using individual-level constructs to work toward a parsimonious model of individual and system change.

Determinants of Intervention Process and Outcome. We argue from example for the importance of recognizing that the factors of intervention content, participant, provider, and setting all are major determinants of intervention outcome and therefore targets for change and candidates for measurement. Our recent review of the smoking prevention literature (Best and others, 1988) provides fragmentary empirical support for this concept. The literature on psychotherapy research provides a clear parallel, showing that variables of these kinds interact to determine outcome. It comes as no surprise to those steeped in program evaluation traditions to realize that we are likely to be more productive if, instead of merely asking what type of program content is most effective, we also ask what type of program works with what type of person and how the success of the program varies across settings and in the hands of different providers. Somewhat surprisingly, these issues have not been addressed seriously in the health promotion field.

Stages of Change. We already have seen how the time dimension affects conceptualization of outcomes. At the individual level, research shows how targets and processes of change differ as a function of readiness. The four steps in diffusion illustrate a similar *process* perspective on intervention impacts at the systems level.

A process conceptualization of outcomes is fundamentally important to the design of health promotion evaluations. We rarely appreciate the implications fully. For example, smoking onset has been described as taking place over a two-year period (Leventhal and Cleary, 1980), while smoking cessation occurs over an average of seven years (Prochaska, Velicer, DiClemente, and Fava, 1988). Multiple interventions occur, both planned and unplanned. During this time, there is an evolution toward a change from nonsmoking to smoking, or vice versa. However, evaluators rarely track this process in its entirety. Instead, we take "snapshots" at a particular point in time and arbitrarily call this the outcome.

To understand the importance of the process perspective more fully, we must recognize that behavioral change is not linear and tidy. Instead, initial change efforts are most often unsuccessful (Prochaska and others, 1985). Individuals (and systems) are changed by the intervention process, but the outcome typically is not the behavioral change intended by the program; rather, it is a smaller step toward ultimate change. The "unsuccessful changers" may revert to an earlier stage and try again, perhaps in response to the next intervention (planned or unplanned) that reaches them. How, then, should we conceptualize the outcome of a specific, time-limited intervention program? We suggest that the ideal way is to approximate with our designs and measures the naturally occurring processes we hope to change. In practice, we compromise of necessity, considering study aims and resources.

Influences on Choice and Treatment of Outcome Measures

We have been arguing for a three-dimensional perspective on conceptualizing health promotion outcomes. The health promotion research, development, and diffusion sequence typically begins when one tries to initiate change at the individual level. Even at this level, change outcomes are best seen as parts of an ongoing process, rather than as discrete events or states. As health promotion progresses toward diffusion, there is an increasing need to conceptualize interventions and outcomes at the systems level. The provider and setting factors become more salient. Intervention becomes more complex and multilayered, including both the originally conceived intervention and the system changes necessary for its diffusion.

This perspective raises a number of new concerns for the design and analysis of health promotion research. The remainder of this chapter will spell out some of the key questions to address, with emphasis on their implications for conceptualizing outcomes.

Theoretical and Conceptual Issues

Linking Outcomes to Intervention Levels. How should the intervention be applied? Depending on the nature of the intervention and the stage of research, we may choose to intervene at the individual level (for example, one-to-one counseling for smoking cessation) or at a system or cluster level (for example, classroom-based education programs). As we move toward diffusion, intervention elements may be applied at multiple levels. For example, in a comprehensive community intervention, the intervention elements may be directed at the population level (for example, mass media), at subsystems (for example, schools and worksites), or at individuals (for example, physicians who offer smoking cessation counseling). Intervention at multiple levels is presumed to produce synergistic effects. If multiple interventions are occurring simultaneously, and if the different levels of intervention influence one another, how are outcomes to be assessed and attributed to specific intervention elements? The use of single-subject designs (for example, multiple baseline) may be generalized from the individual to the organizational or community levels; such designs may help to disentangle these complex relationships (see McKillip, this volume).

Linking Outcomes to Stage of Change. Consider the stages of smoking onset. We may choose to intervene when the target population is at the preparation stage (for example, in elementary school), the initiation stage (for example, in junior high school), or the maintenance stage (for example, in high school or at the university or first job). The outcome measure will be different at each stage. At the initiation stage, for example, differences in behavioral intentions, or in the proportion of students experimenting at the end of grade eight, would be appropriate outcomes. With a high school–based intervention, regular smoking at the end of grade twelve, or cessation rate, might be more appropriate. From the diffusion perspective, analogous measures may well be estimated and used as outcome measures (for example, intention to adopt, actual adoption rates, and long-term maintenance rates).

Length of Follow-up Period. For how long should subjects be followed? Ideally, we would intervene and then follow the study population until the ultimate disease end point was seen. For most health promotion studies, however, only behavioral outcomes are feasible, but we usually do not have the resources even to follow study participants to the ultimate behavioral endpoint. In studies of smoking prevention, for example, reduced rates of experimentation observed at age thirteen have been extrapolated to infer reduced rates of regular smoking at age seventeen. If onset is only *delayed* by the intervention, serious problems with accurate assessment of the intervention's power will occur. Similarly, in diffusion studies, will it follow that differences in rate of adoption at three years will predict different rates of adoption farther down the line?

Design and Measurement Issues

Method of Assignment. At the early stages of research and development, subjects often are randomized to conditions and tracked over time, to allow a fine-grained analysis of the intervention process. However, as we progress through the sequence toward diffusion, population-based studies will have better internal and external validity with the random assignment of intact clusters of individuals (for example, classes, schools, or communities). This has implications for sample size calculations and data analysis because intact clusters will tend to behave more similarly than will independent individuals (see Koepke and Flay, this volume).

Control/Comparison Group. What is the nature of the control/comparison group? In therapeutic intervention trials, individuals are randomly assigned to control groups, and methods to ensure that individuals and/or providers are blind to group membership are strictly enforced. In particular, considerable care is taken to avoid contamination of control subjects. As health promotion research progresses through the stages outlined here, it becomes progressively more difficult to avoid contamination. Health promotion programs can be developed by interested persons in control sites and implemented, even if not in the most efficient manner. Contamination from the popular press, mass media, and so forth, is difficult to control. The implications of such contamination for sample size calculations need to be considered in study design. If the relevant study outcome is to be assessed over the long term, the effect of changing population norms must also be assessed.

Range of Measures. We want to measure important sources of variance in program outcomes. If the design compares one or more intervention contents (for example, social influences versus health facts curricula), these important sources of variance will include participant, provider, and setting variables. Changes in one area influence changes in the others. Because outcomes are often "chained," some may be outcome (dependent) variables early in the process and explanatory (independent) variables later. The stage of the research, the nature of the research question, and the information needed to plan the anticipated next step will determine how broad a range of variables to include, as well as which ones will serve as the primary focus.

Data Sources. Who or what should be observed? Who should provide verbal reports? Study participants will need to be assessed if the actual behavioral outcomes are of primary importance. However, if adoption or diffusion is a primary study interest, then data from persons responsible for adopting the intervention will be needed, as well as data about barriers to diffusion. These data will be used to calculate the rate and quality of diffusion. Unobtrusive measures (for example, time sampling to determine the rate of use of cigarette vending machines or the proportion of restaurants with ashtrays) may be especially useful in evaluating change at a systems level.

Accuracy. Issues of reliability and validity need to be considered. For example, in a smoking prevention study focusing on a behavioral outcome, we need to be sure that students can and will provide accurate information on use or non-use of tobacco, and on the amount used. Biochemical validation for a randomly selected subset of participants may validate self-reports, and provide a basis for estimating self-report error. As another example, we may suspect that "setting" variables such as teacher behaviors will directly influence quality of program implementation, but what is the best way to retrieve that information? (For instance, can principals provide reliable and valid data on smoking rates among teachers?)

Longitudinal Versus Cross-Sectional Designs. The reality that health-related behavioral change occurs over a long period of time presents a fundamental design choice. In medical clinical trials, subjects are followed longitudinally, and changes in health status are observed at the individual level. At the early stages of health promotion research, this strategy may also be feasible. It has the advantage of facilitating process analysis but can be costly and difficult to implement because of the need to track, locate, and measure individual subjects. When the intervention is to be studied at the population level, repeated cross-sectional studies may be more cost-effective. However, it is difficult to relate population changes to changes in individual factors when one is using data of this type. The cross-sectional strategy also needs to account for sample biases that may be introduced by the program. For example, interventions that focus on teen pregnancy reduction may also encourage pregnant girls to stay in school; the result may be a higher count of in-school pregnant girls and hence an apparent (mistaken) increase in pregnancies across the cross-sectionally sampled cohorts.

Frequency of Measurement. How frequently should measures be taken? To study process effectively, it is important to measure frequently at times when change is expected to be rapid. In smoking cessation studies, for example, frequent assessments early in the process, and less frequent assessments later, will provide better process data than will assessments spaced equally over time. Identification of probable key points in the process is essential to adequate definition of a measurement system.

Analysis Issues

Distribution. What are the distributional properties of the measure? When measuring harmful behaviors, we often obtain a large number of individuals reporting no occurrences (for example, no cigarettes smoked in the past week), with the remainder reporting a number of occurrences that follow a distribution that is (often) positively skewed. We actually often hope for a "zero heavy" distribution if the intervention is successful. Standard regression, analysis of variance, and other models that assume normally distributed scores may not be appropriate in this situation. Similarly, categorical measures sensitive to the stage of change require analysis methods that deal specifically with ordered categorical variables. Methods for dealing with longitudinal data on binary outcomes and ordered categorical variables have only recently been developed (for example, see Zeger, Liang, and Self, 1985; Stram, Wei, and Ware, 1988).

Validity of Summary Statistics. Does the method of data summary and analysis create problems for interpretation? For example, consider the "zero heavy" distributions just described. If we report an average number of occurrences as a summary statistic, we do not differentiate between a group with many zeros and a few heavy smokers, on the one hand, and a group with few zeros and many moderate smokers, on the other. We may conclude that there is no difference between the groups, when in fact the outcome for the second group may be far worse since moderate use increases the probability of higher levels of use in the future.

Level and Covariables. Our intervention model assumes that we may obtain covariables at the individual, cluster, and/or higher systems levels. We may need methods of analysis that can model the effects of covariables at all levels while also modeling correlations between individuals within groups. In addition, in attempting to understand change-process issues and outcomes and how the intervention may mediate this process, we need to use methods for handling covariables that change with time.

Model of Outcome Process. What is a reasonable model for the change process in question? For example, if we measure the number of school districts adopting a curriculum and attempt to relate this measure to diffusion factors, should we assume that all districts would adopt the curriculum if they received a large enough diffusion "dose"? Or would a more reasonable model be that a certain proportion of the school districts are "immotive" and will never adopt the curriculum, while the others will adopt it, given an intervention that is appropriate with respect to content, timing, and "dose"? The method of analysis will differ in the two situations.

Data Limitations. How does the analysis deal with incomplete data on the process? In either repeated cross-sectional surveys or longitudinal studies with fixed periods of assessment, information relevant to process questions is incomplete. For example, we may know that an individual is in the maintenance stage now; but with repeated cross-sectional data, the stage at the previous time of ascertainment will be unknown or perhaps unreliably known because of problems of recall. Similarly, with longitudinal data, the individual's stage may be known at each end point of an interval when data are collected, but the number of transitions from one stage to another within the interval may not be known. In either case, modeling of the transition between the stages can be complicated.

Conclusion

We have tried to achieve two aims in this chapter. First, we have shown that conceptualization of health promotion outcomes is anything but simple. The conceptual model changes as we move through the sequence of research, development, and diffusion. Second, if we take the point of view that outcome is best conceptualized as a process, the implications for design, measurement, and analysis are profound. Just as clinical epidemiology started to be seen two decades ago as the science of clinical medicine, so do we need a conceptual framework and methodology to guide applications of behavioral science principles and knowledge to research, development, and diffusion in health promotion.

References

Abrams, D. B., Elder, J. P., Carleton, R. A., Lasater, T. M., and Artz, L. M. "Social Learning Principles for Organizational Health Promotion: An Integrated Approach." In M. F. Cataldo and T. J. Coates (eds.), *Health and Industry: A Behavioral Medicine Perspective.* New York: Wiley, 1986.

Ajzen, I., and Fishbein, M. *Understanding Attitudes and Predicting Social Behavior.* Englewood Cliffs, N.J.: Prentice-Hall, 1980.

Bandura, A. *Social Foundations of Thought and Action: A Social Cognitive Theory.* Englewood Cliffs, N.J.: Prentice-Hall, 1986.

44

Best, J. A. "Intervention Perspectives on School Health Promotion Research." *Health Education Quarterly*, in press.

Best, J. A., Thomson, S. J., Santi, S., Smith, E. A., and Brown, K. S. "Preventing Cigarette Smoking Among School Children." *Annual Review of Public Health*, 1988, *9*, 161–201.

Best, J. A., Wainwright, P. E., Mills, D. E., and Kirkland, S. A. "Biobehavioral Approaches to Smoking Control." In W. Linden (ed.), *Biological Barriers in Behavioral Medicine*. New York: Plenum, 1988.

Blackburn, H., Luepker, R. V., Kline, F. G., Bracht, N., Carlaw, R., Jacobs, D., Mittelmark, M., Stauffer, L., and Taylor, H. L. "The Minnesota Heart Health Program: A Research and Demonstration Project in Cardiovascular Disease Prevention." In J. D. Matarazzo, S. M. Weiss, J. A. Herd, N. E. Miller, and S. M. Weiss (eds.), *Behavioral Health: A Handbook of Health Enhancement and Disease Prevention*. New York: Wiley, 1984.

Chassin, L., Presson, C. C., and Sherman, S. J. "Cigarette Smoking and Adolescent Psychosocial Development." *Basic and Applied Social Psychology*, 1984, *5*, 295–315.

Farquhar, J. W., Fortmann, S. P., Maccoby, N., Wood, P. D., Haskell, W. L., Taylor, C. B., Flora, J. A., Solomon, D. S., Rogers, T., Adler, E., Breitrose, P., and Weiner, L. "The Stanford Five-City Project: An Overview." In J. D. Matarazzo, S. M. Weiss, J. A. Herd, N. E. Miller, and S. M. Weiss (eds.), *Behavioral Health: A Handbook of Health Enhancement and Disease Prevention*. New York: Wiley, 1984.

Flay, B. R. "Efficacy and Effectiveness Trials (and Other Phases of Research) in the Development of Health Promotion Programs." *Preventive Medicine*, 1986, *15*, 451–474.

Greenwald, P., and Cullen, J. W. "The Scientific Approach to Cancer Control." *CA: A Cancer Journal for Physicians*, 1985, *10*, 328–332.

Lasater, T. M., Abrams, D. B., Artz, L. M., Beaudin, P., Cabrera, L., Elder, J., Ferreira, A., Knisley, P., Peterson, G., Rodrigues, A., Rosenberg, P., Snow, R., and Carleton, R. A. "Lay Volunteer Delivery of a Community-Based Cardiovascular Risk Factor Change Program: The Pawtucket Experiment." In J. D. Matarazzo, S. M. Weiss, J. A. Herd, N. E. Miller, and S. M. Weiss (eds.), *Behavioral Health: A Handbook of Health Enhancement and Disease Prevention*. New York: Wiley, 1984.

Leventhal, H., and Cleary, P. D. "The Smoking Problem: A Review of the Research and Theory in Behavioral Risk Modification." *Psychological Bulletin*, 1980, *88*, 370–405.

National Heart, Lung, and Blood Institute. *Guidelines for Demonstration and Education Research Grants*. Washington, D.C.: National Heart, Lung, and Blood Institute, 1983.

Pechacek, T. "A Randomized Trial for Smoking Cessation." Paper delivered to the Sixth World Conference on Smoking and Health, Tokyo, Japan, 1987.

Perry, C. L., Klepp, K-I., and Sillers, C. "Community-Wide Strategies for Cardiovascular Health: The Minnesota Heart Health Program Youth Program." *Health Education Research*, in press.

Perry, C. L., Luepker, R. V., Murray, D. M., and Hearn, M. D. "Parent Involvement with Children's Health Promotion: A One-Year Follow-Up of the Minnesota Home Team." *Health Education Quarterly*, in press.

Prochaska, J., DiClemente, C., Velicer, W., Ginpil, S., and Norcross, J. "Predicting Change in Smoking Status for Self-Changers." *Addictive Behaviors*, 1985, *10*, 407–412.

Prochaska, A., Velicer, W., DiClemente, C., and Fava, J. "Measuring Processes of Change: Applications to the Cessation of Smoking." *Journal of Consulting and Clinical Psychology*, 1988, *56*, 520–528.

Stram, D. O., Wei, L. J., and Ware, J. H. "Analysis of Repeated Ordered Categorical Outcomes with Possibly Missing Observations and Time-Dependent Covariates." *Journal of the American Statistical Association*, 1988, *83*, 631–637.

Zeger, S. L., Liang, K., and Self, S. G. "The Analysis of Binary Longitudinal Data with Time-Independent Covariates." *Biometrika*, 1985, *72*, 31–38.

J. Allan Best is a professor in the Department of Health Studies at the University of Waterloo and director of the Waterloo Smoking Projects, all of which build on the research-development-diffusion model described here.

K. Stephen Brown is a professor in the Department of Statistics and Actuarial Science at the University of Waterloo, codirector of the Waterloo Smoking Projects, and director of the Statistical Consulting Service.

Roy Cameron is the chair of the Health Studies Department and a coinvestigator on the two major Waterloo Smoking Projects.

Edward A. Smith is an assistant professor of health studies and a coinvestigator on the two major Waterloo Smoking Projects.

Marjorie MacDonald directs field operations for the Waterloo Smoking-Prevention Project and previously directed the Waterloo Correspondence Weight-Control Project.

A critical multiplism evaluation approach guided the design, implementation, and assessment of a psychoeducational intervention for surgical patients.

Uses of Evaluation in a Program to Promote Recovery from Surgery

Frederica W. O'Connor, Thomas D. Cook, Elizabeth C. Devine

The traditional patient role encourages hospital patients to be passive, the willing conformers to complex and unfamiliar hospital routines directed by a bewildering array of hospital personnel. There is reason to believe that this uninformed, passive state often retards recovery, perhaps because surgery and hospitalization are unnecessarily appraised as overwhelming (Lazarus and Launier, 1978), leading to high levels of anxiety (Lazarus and Averill, 1972) and other negative emotions that have been widely associated with adverse health consequences (Kimball, 1977). It would presumably be advisable if patients were better informed about what was going to happen to them and why, if they were successfully encouraged to ask questions about their therapy, if they felt free to reach out for help, if they knew about actions they could take themselves to promote their recovery, and if they were encouraged to perform such

The authors would like to acknowledge the many seasons of intellectual collaboration with and mutual encouragement from their colleagues that made possible the several interlocking phases of the work described in this chapter.

Marc T. Braverman (ed.). *Evaluating Health Promotion Programs.*
New Directions for Program Evaluation, no. 43. San Francisco: Jossey-Bass, Fall 1989.

actions. This chapter reports on the design and evaluation of a workshop to help nurses provide psychoeducational care that teaches and helps surgical patients to take an active role in their own recovery from surgery. Particular attention is paid to the many different functions evaluation played in designing and evaluating the workshop, for we believe evaluation has rarely been used in so many self-conscious ways to promote program design.

The starting point for the research was a meta-analysis of 102 studies, which showed that a focused psychoeducational intervention reduced by one-and-a-half days the length of hospital stay of surgical patients and enhanced other clinically relevant outcomes, such as the amount of pain medication taken (Devine and Cook, 1983, 1986). Examination of the studies in the meta-analysis revealed that psychoeducation typically includes some combination of three dimensions. The *information* dimension involves apprising patients of the likely course of their treatment and of the timing and rationale for particular events. Patients are also encouraged to ask questions about hospital procedures, on the assumption that this reduces any anxiety patients may be experiencing. The second dimension involves teaching patients certain *skills* that reduce postoperative complications and give a sense of control. These skills are turning, deep breathing, coughing, and leg and foot exercises. The third dimension is *social support*. Patients are encouraged to seek assistance from the nursing staff and family, with the nurses providing reassurance and assistance with problem solving and coping.

The meta-analysis revealed a salient limitation of the existing data base in that hospital staff administered the intervention in only four of the 102 studies examined. These studies showed fewer positive patient improvements than those in which researchers delivered the intervention. Since financially squeezed hospitals are not likely to hire additional personnel to provide psychoeducational care, our overall goal in the research presented here was to develop and evaluate a treatment designed to sharpen this ability in surgical staff nurses. More specifically, we wanted to specify an optimally effective protocol for psychoeducational care, implement a transferable in-service program that might facilitate the nurses' consistent use of the protocol, evaluate nurses' delivery of the protocol, and assess patient outcomes.

What Is Effective Psychoeducational Care, and How Did Evaluation Help Us Determine It?

The first step in developing an intervention is to arrive at a clear and justifiable definition of the content domain. Our meta-analytical work revealed that the size of the treatment effect increased with the number of dimensions included in an intervention. An examination of the correlations between the effect sizes and more molecular intervention elements within each dimension permitted us to discover the elements within each dimension that were associated with larger effects, further helping us define what a particularly effective intervention might be. While we demonstrated through stratification analyses that effect sizes did not depend on whether a study was published or on whether it used random assignment, we obviously did not "remove" the cumulative effects of all such forces. Consequently, because analysis of the effectiveness of individual intervention elements may have been confounded with study-level characteristics, the meta-analysis does not permit claiming with any certainty that individual elements were causally linked to outcomes. However, the meta-analysis made a crucial contribution to the development of a presumably powerful protocol listing the full range of effective intervention elements.

Two of the authors have been practicing nurses, and our clinical experience was used to edit the quantitative results into a practical package. Since any protocol has to meet the particular needs of hospitals contemplating its use, we visited the hospital in which we were to intervene, discussing the proposed protocol with nursing administrators and spending many months observing the behavior of staff nurses. Once the protocol was determined from the meta-analysis, our professional experience as nurses, and our knowledge of the implementing hospital, an issue arose: How could we make the protocol available to staff nurses, so that they would be willing and able to implement it as part of their routine practice?

What Makes an Effective Workshop, and How Did Evaluation Theory and Practice Help Us Construct One?

When the objective is to incorporate significant new behaviors into ongoing practice, it is not enough to teach the content outlined in a protocol. It is also necessary to prepare clinicians for any organizational and environmental factors that may influence treatment integrity. Thus, the design of a workshop has to incorporate not only a valid program theory (as our development of the protocol tried to accomplish) but also a theory of implementing the protocol. We therefore examined four empirically based theories of implementation, whose central premises are briefly described below.

Implementation Theories. Bardach (1977) views implementation as a complex assembly process that requires coordinating many actors, all pursuing agendas that are not necessarily compatible with one another or with the requirements of a new program. Conflicts between personal and program agendas hinder the assembly process. Obstacles of a less personal nature can also bedevil implementation; for example, the available resources may fail to coincide with program needs, or the program theory may simply be wrong. Because it is impossible to foresee all implementation problems, Bardach recommends designating a "fixer"—a person or a committee with broad access to information about a program and with the power to take remedial actions. Given Bardach's theory, we analyzed the nurses' and administrators' latent agendas, addressed in the workshop the more salient areas of lack of correspondence between them, and proposed ourselves as partial fixers to whom the nurses could turn to discuss implementation issues for six months after the workshop. For difficulties that were more fundamental and required a formal organizational response, we discussed the problems and specific remedial actions with head nurses.

Williams's (1980) managerial theory of implementation holds that the commitment of managers is crucial to ensuring good implementation. Once commitment is achieved and communicated, the central tasks are then to minimize complexity and contradictory demands at the service-delivery level and to develop the capabilities of all personnel, so that they can respond independently and effectively when unforeseen difficulties arise, as they inevitably will. In Williams's view, communication should be nonauthoritarian, inducing cooperation by providing practical guidance for action. In light of Williams's recommendations, we ensured that nursing administrators committed resources to the workshop and clearly expressed their support for it to staff nurses. In the workshop, we acknowledged the implementation predicaments that nurses who are already overworked confront. To reduce the complexity and contradictory demands on nurses, we explored with them ways to build better psychoeducational care into their existing practice, rather than adding another class of care to their already crowded work day.

In Berman's (1978) contingency theory, successful implementation depends on intricate and only partly predictable interactions among various characteristics of the innovation, the setting, and the implementation strategies. No single generic approach to implementation is possible, and in any single case the best approach is likely to be a tailored blend of programmed and adaptive activities (Berman, 1980; Berman and Pauly, 1975). We quickly learned that any implementation strategy in the target hospital had to be built around two salient contingencies. First, nurses prefer learning by doing, rather than by hearing lectures. Second, they are accustomed to considerable autonomy in their interactions with patients. Thus, Berman's theory led us to frame the psychoeducational protocol as a guideline and not as a blueprint, emphasizing that nurses should be free to identify their own strategies for effectively implementing the protocol. Berman's theory also contributed to our decision to divide the workshop into two parts, leaving the second session open for discussion of any implementation obstacles (and solutions) that nurses independently identified after the first workshop session and before the second one.

Fullan (1982) asserts that practitioners' interpretation of how a new practice will affect the daily work routine largely determines the degree to which an innovation is successfully implemented. After surveying the implementation research in education, Fullan concluded that high-quality implementation occurs when practitioners regard a proposed change as needed, when they are clear about its goals and the paths to achieving the goals, when the change is substantial enough to require a reassessment of past practice, and when high-quality materials are available. Organizational characteristics that portend success are prior success with innovations, careful preparation for the implementation process, and staff development that provides interactive experiences to work through new conceptualizations, skills, or behaviors. At the work-group level, managerial support, collegial open exchange, and self-efficacy predict implementation success. Fullan's theory buttressed our decision to schedule the workshop in two parts and to encourage discussion and even disagreement in order to get nurses to confront frankly and work through any hesitations they had about the importance and feasibility of the practices and philosophy we were proposing.

We relied heavily on these four implementation theorists in designing the workshop, but their work was not sufficient. Although they distilled the wisdom from past inquiries into success and failure in implementing social programs, their recommendations were not specific enough for the particular hospital in which the psychoeducational practices were to be implemented. Another source of information was needed, and we turned from generalized theory to site-specific data collection.

The Preworkshop Questionnaire. The review of the implementation literature led us to develop a list of factors that could facilitate or impede the implementation of effective psychoeducational care in the particular hospital we were studying. On a questionnaire distributed before the workshop, nurses were asked to indicate the extent to which each of these factors influenced the quality of the psychoeducational care they already gave routinely. Responses to these items allowed us to identify what nurses expected to be difficult about implementation, helping us identify ways to counteract these potential impediments. Thus, an evaluative questionnaire complemented the literature review, helping us structure the workshop design.

The Workshop. The workshop itself consisted of two ninety-minute sessions conducted about four weeks apart and undertaken with nurses from two general surgery units of a university-affiliated suburban hospital. Each session was repeated six times to accommodate the schedules of all registered nurses who worked more than eight hours per week. All eligible nurses were fully trained.

The first session was designed to acquaint nurses with the treatment protocol and to motivate them to use it by sensitizing them to the benefits usually resulting from upgraded psychoeducational care. We provided feedback on the level and quality of care in their hospital and on the specific elements of practice most in need of improvement, as assessed from six months of previous data collection. This identified for the nurses the specific areas where, in the aggregate, there were particularly large discrepancies between what they were already providing and what the new protocol required of them, counteracting any tendency the nurses might have had to believe, "We already do that." Next, the nurses discussed a videotape of a nurse giving psychoeducational care to a surgery patient and the patient responding to the care (Cook and Cook, 1987). The videotape gave nurses one specific model of how to improve practice, although we stressed that the protocol should be tailored by each nurse to suit individual patient considerations, including different diagnoses.

The second workshop session was devoted to nurses' experiences in trying to implement the workshop protocol. The objective was to let nurses tell us of any difficulties they had encountered in implementing the protocol and to let them share with us and their colleagues any solutions they had worked out for themselves. All this served to reinforce the idea that implementation problems are a normal part of change and that not all such problems can be foreseen. The nurses reported no difficulty in knowing what to do, but they overwhelmingly identified lack of time as the major problem hindering high-quality implementation. An additional problem identified by the researchers was the lack of any formal organizational rewards for psychoeducational care. A list of individual-level, unit-level, and organizational-level solutions for each of the identified problems was compiled from the discussions and subsequently discussed with nursing administrators.

What Makes an Effective Analysis of Implementation, and How Did Evaluation Practice and Theory Help?

The design we used for studying whether the workshop increased implementation involved contrasting the care given after the workshop with that given before the workshop. We used three types of patients and three measures of implementation. Each of the measures evaluated information, skills training, and components of social support.

Cholecystectomy patients were presented as the exemplar group in the workshop, but we stressed that the protocol was broadly applicable. To evaluate whether the workshop increased the level of psychoeducational care provided, we collected data from patients with cholecystectomies, patients with other types of abdominal surgery, and patients with transurethral resections of the prostate (TURP). The last two populations were used not only to assess whether the nurses generalized any of the novel psychoeducational behaviors to nonexemplar patient groups but

also to assess whether any increases in the time devoted to cholecystectomy patients decreased the level of care provided to the nontargeted
patient groups.

The three modes of measurement were patients' reports, nurse observations, and nurses' reports. We describe the measures below and discuss
why such a multimethod approach to measurement was required.

Patients' Reports. All patients in the preworkshop cohort had been
discharged before the beginning of the workshops, and postworkshop
patient recruitment was not initiated until all nurses had attended the
first workshop session. Patients were typically telephoned on the day
after discharge and were asked a series of questions about the care they
had received. Interviews during their hospital stays were not considered
desirable because interaction with researchers at that time may have influenced how the patients interacted with staff nurses. Moreover, telephone
interviews reduced but did not eliminate the possibility that the nonverbal
behavior of interviewers, who knew when the workshop was offered,
might lead to spurious preworkshop-postworkshop differences. The interviews covered all the skills and most of the psychosocial support concepts
in the psychoeducational care protocol. However, to keep the interviews
under thirty minutes, items were asked about only six broad areas in the
information domain.

Patients' reports are advantageous for assessing the delivery of psychoeducational care because a relatively large patient sample can be
recruited, and the questions can tap into all aspects of care that patients
can reasonably be expected to remember. However, several caregivers provide psychoeducational interventions to hospitalized patients, who may
not be able to differentiate among them later. Thus, patients' reports
have the drawback of being unable to link particular teaching to particular nurses. They are also problematic if patients cannot fully recall what
occurred during a stressful time some days earlier, or if general satisfaction with their treatment causes patients to recall what happened with
a positive halo. Although any of these biases may have operated, the
present study is about *changes* in implementation levels. Thus, the threat
to be controlled for is differential bias at each time, and it is difficult to
imagine why any bias may have differed between the preworkshop and
postworkshop cohorts. Useful as patients' reports are, they do not constitute a perfect measure of psychoeducational care, and so our critical
multiplist approach to measurement (Cook, 1985) inclined us to add
other measures with different limitations.

Nurse Observations. Twenty nurses were observed for a single eight-
hour shift by either of two researchers, both two or three months before
the workshop and three or four months after the workshop. Data were
collected about a comprehensive set of elements from the information,
skills, and social support dimensions. Observations were chosen as the

second mode of data collection because they permit a comprehensive picture of the psychoeducational behaviors nurses actually perform throughout a shift. They also make it possible to identify other forces in the setting that make demands on nurses' attention, and since events are recorded as they occur, faulty recall is not an issue.

However, observations in this case had their drawbacks. First, the observers were salient, and nurses may have upgraded their psychoeducational care because of this. Second, the observers knew when the workshop occurred and may have rated differently at the pre- and postworkshop observations. Third, the observations were based on individual practitioners' interactions with patients during an eight-hour period, but the same patients may have received psychoeducational care from other practitioners on that same shift, when the observer was not present. Fourth, the sample of patients was small, and there were many variance-inducing irrelevancies associated with other demands on nurses' time. Fifth, several nurses were dropped from the analysis because they did not care for a qualifying patient at both the pre- and postworkshop observation periods. Instability would be reduced by a more extensive sampling plan that could generate observations involving more nurses, more patients, and more work shifts. Because direct observations are so expensive and time-consuming, however, we had to accept the heterogeneity, the small number of cases, and the consequent low level of statistical power; otherwise, we would not have had much understanding of the contexts in which nurses' behavior occurred.

Nurses' Reports. The final mode of data collection was nurses' reports. Questionnaires were distributed to nurses one month before the workshop and seven months later, when all the outcome data had been collected. The questionnaires contained sixty-seven items from the three dimensions making up psychoeducational care, and nurses estimated the proportion of typical abdominal patients for whom they provided a particular element of care each month. These reports permitted efficient collection of a large amount of information, but at the cost of an apparent social desirability bias (for a discussion of self-report measures, see D'Onofrio, this volume; Scheirer and Rezmovic, 1983).

Results

Changes in Psychoeducational Care. As expected, the absolute levels of psychoeducational care differed by measure across both the preworkshop and postworkshop measurements, with nurses' reports being invariably the highest. However, our key hypothesis was about *changes* in implementation, and we found a high degree of consistency when we aggregated across the three patient types and compared the direction of pretest-posttest changes. For the information dimension, increases were observed for all three modes, although only the results for patients' reports were statistically reliable. For the skills domain, postworkshop means were slightly higher than preworkshop means for each method, although none was statistically reliable. For psychosocial support, a reliable increase was registered on the patients' reports and a small nonreliable increase on the full-shift observations, although the nurses' reports showed a reliable decrease in psychosocial support. This was the only anomalous finding in an otherwise congruent pattern. In eight cases out of nine, the level of psychoeducational care was higher after the workshop than before (O'Connor and others, 1989).

Providing more patient care to the targeted cholecystectomy patients did not lead nurses to neglect other patients, for results similar to those found for the targeted patients were also obtained for the other abdominal patients and the TURP patients. Further, nurses did not neglect other areas of nursing care as they increased psychoeducation, for postworkshop ratings were higher for all three satisfaction items, despite preworkshop ratings close to a ceiling effect. The nurses' reports gave a clue to why this happened. Those data showed that nurses believed they were able to provide more psychoeducational care primarily because they provided it simultaneously with physical care, instead of as an add-on.

Patient Outcomes. The length of hospital stay for patients in the experimental sample reliably decreased between the pretest and posttest. More important, this occurred when experimental patients were compared to similar patients from a nearby control hospital owned by the same corporation; 65 percent of the patients in the sample were treated by surgeons who operated at both hospitals. Use of antinausea and sleep medications also decreased by reliably more in the experimental hospital. While changes in analgesic use were less clear, they were also in the predicted direction (Devine and others, 1988).

Did the Workshop "Cause" Implementation to Increase? It is important to assure ourselves that the increases in psychoeducation resulted from the research treatment and not from other factors. One threat to the inference that the workshop *caused* nurses to provide enhanced psychoeducational care is selection, for the preworkshop and postworkshop samples of patients were not formally equivalent (Cook and Campbell, 1979). However, they were compared on many attributes that plausibly could have influenced nurses' psychoeducational care. In no case did the samples differ. Moreover, there were no obvious changes in community makeup or in the delivery of health care during this study. Selection can also be of nurses, as well as of patients. To rule out the possibility that different sets of nurses were included at the pretest and posttest time periods, all the implementation analyses reported here were limited to patients who received preoperative care from those nurses who worked through both the pre- and postworkshop data collection periods (thirty-one of thirty-eight nurses).

A second threat is history—the occurrence of events, other than the research treatment, that may have caused observed effects. The research team had regular contact with nursing management and staff during the study period and noted no activity unrelated to the research that could have increased nurses' psychoeducational care.

A third threat is testing differences between the pre- and postworkshop cohorts. The structured nature of the patient interviews reduced this likelihood, although changes in the interviewers' tone of voice may have differentially biased responses across the cohorts. Differential bias is more plausible with nurse observations. At the first observation, nurses did not know of the behaviors to be targeted in the workshop but were fully informed about them afterward. On the nurses' questionnaire, nurses would have been likely to endorse most elements even before the workshop, but they may have been even more prone to endorse certain items afterward.

Were our results attributable to testers' or nurses' having known for each measure what the research hypotheses differentially demanded from the preworkshop and postworkshop periods? Here, we can refer to the outcome data taken from patients' charts in a pretest-posttest design with a control hospital. Length of stay decreased by more in the experimental hospital than in the control hospital. It is not easy to explain this in terms of the same reporting biases invoked to explain the implementation findings. Why should nurses' and researchers' reporting behavior affect the discharge decisions of physicians? Our inference that the workshop led to increased psychoeducational care is supported not only by the increases in implementation across three patient types but also by a nomological network of relationships that indicate that a higher quality of patient education occurred after the workshop than before (Cronbach and Meehl, 1955).

Conclusion

The research we have just described was successful in getting staff nurses to increase the quality of the psychoeducational care they provided and in getting patients released from the hospital sooner than would otherwise have been the case. We think we have discovered one way to help staff nurses undermine the traditional patient role, with its emphasis on unquestioned compliance and the abrogation of personal control. The psychoeducational approach to care fosters patients' acquisition of knowledge and their perception that they are able to initiate actions that effectively reduce the aversiveness of events and sensations. Being actively involved in their hospital experience not only helps patients but also saves millions of dollars each year in hospital costs.

What was special about the research, from an evaluation perspective, was the large number of evaluation-relevant techniques that were used to design and evaluate the workshop. The meta-analysis led to identification of the components of psychoeducational care most strongly associated with desirable outcomes and hence most worth stressing in an intervention protocol. On-site observations helped us tailor the intervention even more, so as to increase the fit for the hospital in which the demonstration was carried out. Our review of four implementation theories—each in itself a partial product of evaluations of implementation—helped us structure a workshop that was comprehensive and relevant to nurses whose schedules were already too busy. Finally, given the limitations of all single measures, we conducted an evaluation of implementation and outcomes that relied heavily on multiple imperfect measures of both implementation and outcome. The general consistency of outcomes, both within and across related constructs, strengthens the inference that the workshop caused nurses to treat patients differently, which caused patients to recover faster and more easily from surgery.

References

Bardach, E. *The Implementation Game*. Cambridge, Mass.: MIT Press, 1977.

Berman, P. *The Study of Macro and Micro Implementation of Social Policy*. Santa Monica, Calif.: Rand Corporation, 1978.

Berman, P. "Thinking About Programmed and Adaptive Implementation: Matching Strategies to Situations." In H. M. Ingram and D. E. Mann (eds.), *Why Policies Succeed or Fail*. Newbury Park, Calif.: Sage, 1980.

Berman, P., and Pauly, E. W. *Federal Programs Supporting Educational Change*. Vol. 2. *Factors Affecting Change Agent Projects*. Santa Monica, Calif.: Rand Corporation, 1975.

Cook, T. D. "Postpositivist Critical Multiplism." In R. L. Shotland and M. M. Mark (eds.), *Social Science and Social Policy*. Newbury Park, Calif.: Sage, 1985.

Cook, T. D., and Campbell, D. T. *Quasi-Experimentation: Design and Analysis Issues for Field Settings*. Skokie, Ill.: Rand McNally, 1979.

Cook, T. D., and Cook, F. L. *Your Participation in Recovery from Surgery*. Videotape. New York: American Journal of Nursing Co., 1987.

Cronbach, L. J., and Meehl, P. E. "Construct Validity in Psychological Tests." *Psychological Bulletin*, 1955, *52*, 281–302.

Devine, E. C., and Cook, T. D. "A Meta-Analytic Analysis of Psychoeducational Interventions on Length of Postsurgical Hospital Stay." *Nursing Research*, 1983, *32*, 267–274.

Devine, E. C., and Cook, T. D. "Clinical and Cost-Saving Effects of Psychoeducational Interventions with Surgical Patients: A Meta-Analysis." *Research in Nursing and Health*, 1986, *9*, 89–105.

Devine, E. C., O'Connor, F. W., Cook, T. D., Wenk, V. A., and Curtin, T. R. "Clinical and Financial Effects of Psychoeducational Care Provided by Staff Nurses to Adult Surgical Patients in the Post-DRG Environment." *American Journal of Public Health*. 1988, *78*, 1293–1297.

58

Fullan, M. *The Meaning of Educational Change.* New York: Teachers College Press, 1982.

Kimball, C. B. "Psychological Responses to the Experience of Open-Heart Surgery." In R. H. Moos (ed.), *Coping with Physical Illness.* New York: Plenum Press, 1977.

Lazarus, R., and Averill, J. "Emotion and Cognition: With Special Reference to Anxiety." In C. Spielberger (ed.), *Anxiety: Current Trends in Theory and Research.* Vol. 2. Orlando, Fla.: Academic Press, 1972.

Lazarus, R., and Launier, R. "Stress-Related Transactions Between Person and Environment." In L. Pervin and M. Lewis (eds.), *Perspectives in Interactional Psychology.* New York: Plenum Press, 1978.

O'Connor, F. W., Devine, E. C., Cook, T. D., Wenk, V. A., and Curtin, T. R. "Enhancing Implementation of Surgical Nurses' Psychoeducational Care: Effects of a Research-Based Workshop After DRGs." Unpublished manuscript, 1989.

Scheirer, M. A., and Rezmovic, E. L. "Measuring the Degree of Program Implementation: A Methodological Review." *Evaluation Review,* 1983, 7, 283–306.

Williams, W. *The Implementation Perspective.* Berkeley: University of California Press, 1980.

Frederica W. O'Connor is assistant professor of nursing, University of Washington.

Thomas D. Cook is professor of psychology and urban affairs and policy research, Northwestern University.

Elizabeth C. Devine is assistant professor of nursing, University of Wisconsin, Milwaukee.

The use of sensitive self-report data in the evaluation of contemporary health programs raises issues not addressed by textbooks.

The Use of Self-Reports on Sensitive Behaviors in Health Program Evaluation

Carol N. D'Onofrio

The evaluation of many health programs today depends on self-report data about highly sensitive behaviors collected from populations that do not necessarily trust researchers. Evaluating the extent to which a program in AIDS prevention meets its objectives, for example, may require interviewing male homosexuals about the number and nature of their sexual contacts in recent months, their engagement in receptive oral and anal intercourse, and their use of condoms during various sexual activities. Normal reticence about disclosing such intimate information is likely to be heightened in this case by awareness of social sanctions against men with same-gender sexual preferences and by resultant suspicions about how the data will be used. The evaluation design may introduce further complications by requiring that sensitive behavioral information be collected not just once but both before and after program implementation.

In such cases, the information needed for evaluation can be obtained only through self-reports, which are subject to numerous sources of bias. Respondents' concerns about providing the requested information are real, for disclosure of homosexual behavior, for example, has resulted not only in social stigmatization but also in loss of jobs, insurance, and

Marc T. Braverman (ed.). *Evaluating Health Promotion Programs.*
New Directions for Program Evaluation, no. 43. San Francisco: Jossey-Bass, Fall 1989.

housing. The evaluator also may be concerned about his or her ability to keep the data gathered confidential. Controversial proposals for testing and controlling individuals at risk for AIDS could result in forced access to identifying information through court orders or in illegal entry into files. Despite these dangers, obtaining valid behavioral data is critical because the stakes are high. Finding effective preventive approaches is essential to stem the lethal AIDS epidemic. At the same time, AIDS has resulted in so many urgent needs for resources that money cannot be wasted on ineffective efforts. The program evaluator in such a situation faces unprecedented ethical and methodological problems.

The evaluation of programs aimed at preventing alcohol and drug abuse, family violence, teenage pregnancy, sexually transmitted diseases, AIDS in intravenous drug users, and many other health problems also involves substantial reliance on self-reports of sensitive behaviors. A moment's reflection on any one of these topics reveals questions laden with methodological and ethical issues that the evaluator must consider. Will teenagers involved in a school-based program aimed at preventing anorexia and bulimia admit to secretive binge-and-purge eating? Would collecting data about such behavior from a cross-section of students tempt some to try this form of weight control? Will workers whose jobs may be in jeopardy honestly report whether they are following safe procedures for handling toxic substances? Would a regulatory agency use legal means to gain access to such data in order to identify respondents whose unsafe practices create a workplace hazard? Will smokers who have been exposed to an antismoking program admit that they still smoke, when environmental restrictions and mounting social pressure make smoking a subversive activity? Will questioning these persons about their smoking practices be perceived as a source of additional pressure that invades individual rights to privacy and choice?

Textbooks do not address these and other issues raised by the use of sensitive self-report data in the evaluation of contemporary health programs. Designing any such evaluation tests the ingenuity of the researcher in finding new and creative ways to apply established principles and techniques. To assist in this task, this chapter first examines the concept of sensitive behavior and the motives associated with distorted reports of behavior. Against this background, specific ethical issues are discussed and linked to methodological problems in assessing and improving the validity of self-report data. Finally, directions are suggested for strengthening both ethical practice and methodological rigor in health program evaluations.

Sensitive Behavior and Misreporting

Behavior is "sensitive" when it diverges from social norms or when convention dictates that it is too private to be publicly discussed. The sensitivity of a specific behavior varies across cultures and social groups and even within the same group at different times and places. In addition, perceptions about what is sensitive may vary from individual to individual and even for the same individual when the purpose, time, and setting for data collection differ or when different data collection methods are used. This means that the sensitivity of behavior must be assessed within the social context of the respondents to be questioned. Further, methods of data collection are part of that social context.

Since respondents may be reluctant to disclose behaviors considered socially undesirable, and since they may overreport behaving in ways that are socially approved, researchers have long been concerned that behavioral self-reports are biased. Bradburn and Sudman (1979) demonstrate that misreporting increases with the perceived threat of questions about various behavioral topics. These investigators collected data revealing the relative sensitivity of selected behaviors relevant to health. Thus, while only 10 percent of the respondents in a national probability sample indicated that "most people" would be very uneasy about answering questions on drinking, 29 percent believed that most people would be very uneasy about reporting intoxication. More than 56 percent of the respondents felt that most people would be very uneasy about answering questions on masturbation, the most threatening behavior studied.

Behaviors that are the focus of health programs today are likely to be far more sensitive than those investigated by Bradburn and Sudman. Although most such behaviors are likely to be underreported, overreporting may occur under certain circumstances. A closer look at reasons for both types of inaccuracy provides further insight into factors that make behavior sensitive. Such understanding is paramount in addressing ethical issues in data collection and in developing methods to reduce reporting bias.

Reasons for Underreporting Behavior. Respondents are likely to underreport engaging in sensitive behaviors when they perceive that disclosure of accurate information would be risky. The type and strength of the risk anticipated depends on the meaning of the behavior to the individual and on his or her conception of the meanings that others would attribute to it. Gorden (1969) provides a useful discussion of motives for the withholding or underreporting of information in response to sensitive questions, but this analysis must be expanded to encompass the full range of reasons that may lead individuals to distort self-reports of behaviors related to health.

1. *Guilt and denial.* Individuals may feel so guilty or conflicted about behavior that they have difficulty admitting it even to themselves. In such cases, a respondent's conception of the truth is so different from objective reality that survey methods are unlikely to elicit accurate self-report data. Even if respondents are willing to tell the truth, their refer-

ences will be to the truth as they believe it to be, and they will generally be unaware of more objective views (Phillips, 1971). Such denial is commonly associated with alcohol and drug abuse, child abuse, wife battering, and certain eating disorders.

2. *Trauma.* People who have been raped, beaten, or involved in a serious accident may find it painful and acutely unpleasant to discuss their behaviors in conjunction with such events. Questions that force individuals to relive such experiences may be rejected or answered in a perfunctory manner unless discussing them provides catharsis (Gorden, 1969).

3. *Notions about what is personal and private.* Individuals may refuse to cooperate with evaluation studies or may withhold information concerning behaviors that they regard as so private that they are improper to discuss, embarrassing to reveal, or simply no one else's business. Toxic shock syndrome is a recent example of a life-threatening condition that required epidemiological investigators to cross traditional boundaries of privacy in order to collect detailed data about women's personal hygiene practices during menstruation. The most famous example, however, occurred over three decades ago, when Kinsey and his colleagues (1948, 1953) shocked the American public by collecting extensive interview data on sexual behaviors at a time when public talk about sex was restricted to "the vulgar, the moralistic, or the psychoanalytic" (Turner, Miller, and Moses, 1989, p. 79).

4. *Fear of others' reactions.* People may withhold or distort information about their behavior when they fear that full and truthful disclosure would shock the researcher or evoke disapproval. Interviewers' characteristics may affect the type and quality of behavioral information that can be collected. In some cases, respondents may be willing to provide truthful information about their behavior to data collectors, but they fear the reactions of others, should they overhear. Thus, the setting for data collection also can influence the accuracy of self-reports, as illustrated by McKennell's (1980) finding that young boys report a higher incidence of smoking when questioned at school rather than at home.

5. *Fear of social sanctions.* A closely related reason for withholding information about behavior is fear that loss of status or other social sanctions could result if others had access to the self-reported information or if it should become public. People thus may not admit to using illicit drugs, or engaging in violence, because they fear arrest. Those who engage in homosexual or bisexual acts, intercourse outside of marriage, or sex with prostitutes may fear that discovery would threaten their families, employment, or social standing. Since such behaviors are highly sensitive, they may be especially subject to underreporting.

Reasons for Overreporting Behavior. Self-reports of behavior may be biased by overreporting when individuals falsely claim that they engage in certain socially approved behaviors, or that they do so more frequently than is actually the case. Such claims tend to be motivated by respondents' desires to enhance their image, either to themselves or to the data collector. Adolescents eager to appear mature may falsely report that they smoke, use drugs, or engage in sexual intercourse. People of all ages may exaggerate the extent to which they take preventive health actions considered socially desirable (Kristiansen and Harding, 1984). Similarly, physicians have been found to report performing cancer-screening tests more often than medical records indicate they actually do (McPhee, Richard, and Solkowitz, 1986).

Ethical Issues in the Collection and Use of Behavioral Self-Report Data

The application of traditional ethical principles to the collection of behavioral self-reports raises new dilemmas when we consider the character of the behaviors implicated in many of today's health problems and the life circumstances of people whose health is most at risk. As funding agencies, individual investigators, and institutional review boards for the protection of human subjects grapple with issues related to the collection and use of sensitive self-report data, they often differ over specific ethical judgments and the principles on which they are based. Consequently, the health field as a whole currently lacks standards concerning the ethical appropriateness of particular procedures for research and evaluation.

Mounting concerns about ethical issues in sensitive behavioral research involving minors recently led the National Institutes of Health, through the Office for Protection from Research Risks, to convene a working group charged with defining areas of consensus and uncertainty. In exploring largely uncharted ethical territory, this group has identified a number of thorny questions, as a few examples will illustrate. One area of inquiry concerns the extent to which children at different developmental stages understand what they may be revealing and the potential consequences of disclosing information about sensitive behavior. Other complex questions relate to the requirement that parents provide informed consent for children to participate in research. Is parental consent appropriate and feasible when data are to be collected from teenaged mothers, runaways, children whose parents have abused them, or youngsters in foster care? Doubts about the proper limits of confidentiality provide additional illustrations. Can parents legally gain access to sensitive behavioral information that children were assured would be kept confidential? What are the responsibilities of the researcher when young people confidentially reveal that they engage in behaviors which could harm themselves or others?

Equally careful attention is needed in defining and wrestling with ethical issues related to requests for sensitive behavioral information from other special populations. Problem definition and data collection procedures must reflect understanding of cultural differences in the meanings of behavior, contexts in which behavior occurs, and norms for socially acceptable actions. Research with groups who are stigmatized, alienated, and distrustful must reflect sensitivity to the pain of these human conditions.

A cross-cutting ethical question in health-related studies is whether the factors that make a population vulnerable to disease also make it exceptionally vulnerable to risk from disclosing sensitive behavioral information. The poor, minorities, youth, people who know they are at risk for AIDS, those who are caught in the multiple problems associated with chemical dependency, the homeless, and many other groups who are the focus of health programs must struggle constantly to preserve autonomy and ego strength. Since asking the disadvantaged to reveal sensitive information may diminish their autonomy, violate their privacy, and publicly acknowledge their deviation from social norms, collecting such data may be too damaging to justify in the name of health. Listening to sensitive self-reports with a nonjudgmental attitude also may be perceived as sanctioning actions that perpetuate social and health problems. Alternatively, divulging such behavior to a respectful and nonjudgmental listener may have healing potential. Clearly, the risks of harm must be carefully assessed against the direct benefits such populations can expect from participation in evaluation. The very qualities that make behaviors sensitive should sharpen concern about the ethics of collecting self-report data on behavioral performance.

Since motives for misreporting sensitive behaviors reflect conscious or unconscious efforts at self-protection, evidence that self-report data are not valid may reflect respondents' perceptions that the risks of research participation were inadequately controlled or that their rights were inadequately protected. Methods to increase the validity of self-reports in such circumstances must be carefully evaluated against ethical principles. Techniques that even marginally manipulate, deceive, or coerce vulnerable populations in order to obtain more truthful responses may fail to meet ethical standards.

The collection of sensitive behavioral self-reports involves other ethical issues that go beyond concern with the protection of the research participants, for the data obtained shape definitions of the health problem, the population that is at risk, and the preventive actions needed. McDowell and Newell (1987) observe that a given indicator does not serve merely as a passive marker of health but also as a source of influence on social and political goals. Turner, Miller, and Moses (1989) point out that in the absence of good data there is a tendency to use inadequate numbers, even though this involves the serious risk of making wrong predictions and creating the illusion that more is known than is actually known. Other consequences of collecting self-reports on sensitive behaviors in health program evaluations may include unnecessary labeling of sociocultural or racial groups and the definition of certain behaviors as medical problems requiring medical treatment. What is most obvious, of course, is that evaluation results are likely to affect estimates of problem prevalence, the conceptualization of needed interventions, and the fate of health promotion and disease prevention programs. If data are inaccurate, promising programs may be scrapped and ineffective ones disseminated.

Ethical practice in health program evaluation requires valid data and data collection procedures that provide optimum protection and benefit for research participants. This dual requirement inextricably links ethical concerns to methodological issues in the assessment and improvement of the validity of behavioral self-reports.

Assessing the Validity of Self-Report Data

The validity of self-report data is affected by three successive levels of respondents' cooperation: agreement to participate in the study, completion of each question, and truthfulness of responses. Although the latter dimension has dominated the concern over validity of behavioral self-reports in health research, validity also can be compromised by the refusal of individuals to participate in data collection and by their withholding of responses to specific questions.

Rates of refusal to participate in studies of sensitive behavior can be high. In recent research on the sexual experiences of white and Afro-American women in Los Angeles, 45 percent of the women contacted either refused to schedule an interview or terminated telephone recruitment before their eligibility for the survey could be determined (Wyatt, 1988). Such results cast doubt on the representativeness of the sample and therefore on the generalizability of the data obtained. The absence of data on particular questions also threatens external validity. Thus, reviewing existing knowledge about homosexual behavior, Turner, Miller, and Moses (1989) note that about one-quarter of the male respondents in a 1970 national probability sample did not complete the items on same-gender sexual experiences, thereby introducing the possibility of substantial bias in the composition of the sample of men who replied. These examples underscore the importance of sampling issues for estimates of the extent to which self-report data accurately represent the performance of sensitive behaviors in a population.

Assessing the validity of self-report data also poses other problems. Validation requires that the truth be known, but many behaviors that influence health status are known only to the actor. Methods other than self-report for assessing the truth about such behaviors frequently are not available. Published reports of health program evaluations reveal two common responses to this predicament. First, the evaluator may simply proceed with the collection and analysis of self-report data, ignoring the validity issue altogether. Since this approach does not reflect methodological rigor, it does not fulfill the ethical mandate to obtain the most accurate data possible. The second strategy is to attempt validation, but this option also has pitfalls. Various approaches to estimating the truth of self-reports have been tried, but each has methodological limitations. Specific examples are provided by Block (1982) and Midanik (1982) in their reviews of the validity of self-report data concerning, respectively, dietary intake and alcohol consumption.

Direct observation provides the strongest standard against which to validate behavioral self-reports, but many sensitive behaviors are not subject to observation. When observation is feasible, the period covered is likely to be brief, and the researcher cannot be sure that behavior during this interval represents usual behavior. Moreover, a single observer may record an unreliable account of behavior, and unless observation is unobtrusive, awareness of being watched may influence a subject's performance of the behavior under study.

Given these problems, most efforts to validate behavioral self-reports have used another independent measure of behavior as a reference criterion. Many types of evidence from many different sources have been employed. These include collateral reports from friends or relatives, biological or mechanical tests, physiological events, analyses of official records, chronological records kept by the respondent, and, most recently, "garbaeology," or the inspection of household trash (Rabow and Neuman, 1984).

The fundamental problem with this approach to validation is that the independent measures themselves have not been validated against the truth; therefore, they cannot provide a standard for assessing the accuracy of self-reported information. Consequently, the evaluator is faced with the problem of interpreting data about behavior from two different sources, each of which is subject to measurement error. Since the concepts being measured are similar but not identical, the correlations expected and obtained are frequently not high. Moreover, the meaning of these correlations is difficult to interpret, for the theory to explain their relationship is often weak, and there are no clear criteria for determining the degree of association needed to demonstrate adequate validity, even when sophisticated statistical models are used (Turner and Martin, 1984). Correlation coefficients are often simply reported with the conclusion that the criterion measure is valid. This practice has been recognized as a major weakness in validation studies (McDowell and Newell, 1987; Block, 1982).

Testing the validity of a measure against another, independent measure has been termed *concurrent* or *relative validation,* but Block (1982) argues that this approach is more appropriately viewed as *corroboration*. The latter term provides an important reminder to evaluators that the criterion measure, although it may have greater face validity than behavioral self-reports, can also be fallible. Thus, the methodologically rigorous investigator should search for threats to validity, not only in self-report data but also in other behavioral indicators. Further, in interpreting the degree of congruence between behavioral self-reports and independent measures, the assumption should not automatically be made that self-reports are the source of greater error. Miller and Groves (1985) illustrate these principles in their study of official records used to estimate bias in self-reports of victimization. Discovery of numerous weaknesses in the records led these investigators to call for a more complete, standardized procedure for reporting the results of record checks, as well as for a more critical view of findings.

Evaluators also need to recognize that just as psychological, socio-cultural, and situational factors may impair the validity of behavioral self-reports, so may these factors consciously or unconsciously bias the interpretation of behavioral data. Midanik (1982) cautions that alcohol researchers may tend to accept as valid whichever of two measures demonstrates the higher rate of consumption or the worse incidence of problems. Similarly, vested interest in the outcomes of health program evaluation may determine the extent to which self-report data are accepted as valid.

The culture of the health community makes it particularly vulnerable to two sorts of bias in interpreting behavioral evidence. Health researchers socialized in the Western scientific tradition place great value on objective, unbiased data that can be replicated through independent observation. Since behavioral self-reports are subjective, they are inherently unable to satisfy this criterion. Precision of measurement is a related issue, for, as McDowell and Newell (1987) point out, it is by no means self-evident that "soft" subjective data can be considered to be anything more than a crude approximation to measurement. For these reasons, the validity of self-report data is suspect.

Conversely, health scientists often accept biological measures as incontrovertible evidence of behavior. The use of biochemical tests and physiological events to validate behavioral self-reports has been called the "gold standard" of health program evaluation. The collection of biological samples appears to enhance the credibility of evaluation findings—even when specimens are not analyzed! Nevertheless, biomedical indicators are also subject to measurement error, and results can be affected by factors other than behavior. Blood pressure readings, for example, may be influenced by genetic and physiological variables beyond behavioral control. Pregnancy may occur as the result of contraceptive failure. Since biochemical tests vary in sensitivity and specificity, both false positive and false negative results must be expected. The time that a substance remains in the body also limits the time within which biological evidence of certain behaviors can be detected.

Health program evaluators need to familiarize themselves with the technical limitations of biological data and other evidence used to corroborate behavioral self-reports. Potential error should be assessed for all types of measures. Relationships among different data sets should be examined with full consideration of the strengths and weaknesses of the analytical procedures used. While such an approach may still not permit conclusive statements about the validity of sensitive self-reports, the evaluator who applies standards of methodological rigor and intellectual honesty will have provided the strongest possible test.

Improving the Validity of Behavioral Self-Reports

Recognition that the disclosure of sensitive information may be affected by characteristics of data collection instruments and procedures has stimulated many methodological studies. Although the bulk of this work has focused on the expression of opinions and attitudes, in recent years some investigators have examined the influence of methodological factors on the disclosure of sensitive behaviors. For example, after examining the effects of question length and wording familiarity on responses to questions about threatening behaviors, Bradburn and Sudman (1979) recommend separating such questions into two categories: An initial item, requiring only a yes or no response, should inquire whether a behavior was performed even once within some time span, and then the frequency or intensity of the behavior can be established by additional items requiring qualified answers. Methodological research of this nature has led to numerous recommendations for the collection of sensitive self-report data. Following these recommendations may well reduce response error, but several cautions are warranted.

Since methodological research is still continuing, the evaluator should recognize that findings from newer investigations sometimes contradict earlier results on which methodological recommendations have been based. The development and testing of innovations in data collection procedures also may necessitate the revision of previously reached conclusions. For example, the advent of portable computers opens up possibilities for data collection that may lead to more accurate reporting of sensitive behaviors than have the methods previously available (Waterton and Duffy, 1984).

Another illustration can be drawn from experimentation with Warner's (1965) randomized response model. In general, this model involves instructing the respondent to use a randomization device, such as a coin flip or a spinner, to determine whether he or she should answer a sensitive question or an innocuous one. Since the data collector does not know which question has been selected, the respondent's privacy is preserved and, theoretically, his or her willingness to disclose sensitive information is increased. The proportion of respondents who actually do disclose such information is estimated from knowledge about the probability of the sensitive question's having been offered, the sample size, and the proportion of subjects who endorsed the items to which they responded.

Bradburn and Sudman (1979) found that use of the randomized response technique resulted in less distortion of threatening self-reports than did the use of face-to-face and telephone interviews and a self-administered questionnaire. Nevertheless, the latter methods were more effective than the randomized response model in reducing overreporting of socially desirable behavior. This study tested just one version of the model, however, and it is possible that different results would have been obtained if another of its many variations (Carr and Marascuilo, 1982) had been employed.

A larger question is whether results would differ if methodological studies were conducted with other populations or at other times and places. Since the sensitivity of behavior is subject to situational variability, results obtained in one methodological study may not be safely generalized to other research contexts. After experimentally investigating the effects of alternative data collection methods on responses to threatening questions about behavior, Bradburn and Sudman (1979) concluded that accuracy of response by method appears to interact with the population and the behavior being studied.

Yet another caution pertains specifically to program evaluation. Most studies investigating methodological effects on the disclosure of sensitive information involve data collection only, unaccompanied by a program. Consequently, findings do not reflect the possibility that reporting may be influenced by program participation, either alone or in interaction with other variables. Stated somewhat differently, the program itself may create demand characteristics that influence the participant to report behavior consonant with the program's objectives, particularly when data are collected soon after his or her participation in the program ends. More research is needed on the extent to which involvement in a program actually influences behavioral self-reports, as well as on characteristics of programs and participants that may be associated with this source of bias. For example, an individual's identification with the program, its facilitator, or other program participants may increase social expectations for behavior and suppress admissions of noncompliance. Since the dynamics that many health programs foster to facilitate behavioral change also may heighten false reporting of behavior, disentangling these effects represents a difficult methodological challenge in evaluation.

Most methodological recommendations for improving the validity of sensitive self-reports are aimed at increasing respondents' trust and minimizing threat in data collection situations. A conceptually different approach to the enhancement of validity involves informing subjects that the self-reports they provide will be checked against other evidence. This knowledge places respondents in a situation where they must either tell the truth or risk discovery of deception.

Although reference may be made to real data sources, Jones and Sigall (1971) developed a "bogus pipeline" procedure in which experimental subjects were induced to believe that a pseudo lie detector could determine whether responses on a self-administered questionnaire reflected their true attitudes. Evans, Hansen, and Mittelmark (1977) adapted this technique in evaluating a smoking prevention program for youth, and use of the bogus pipeline to enhance the validity of behavioral self-reports is now common in such evaluations. Typically, young people are told that analysis of saliva or expired air samples detects smoking behavior. Biological samples are then collected, and then the young people complete paper-and-pencil questionnaires concerning their smoking behavior. Some studies have found higher reporting when this technique is used, but others have not observed such an effect. Recent research has been directed toward identifying particular conditions under which the bogus pipeline enhances the validity of behavioral self-reports (Murray and Perry, 1987).

The collection of biological samples in this approach is sometimes erroneously referred to as validation, possibly because biological data also can be used to corroborate behavioral self-reports. Such confusion does not advance scientific understanding, and it can even be misleading. Therefore, if evaluators are to avoid deceiving themselves and others, they must clearly distinguish between procedures aimed at increasing the validity of self-reports and those used to assess the validity of data obtained.

Ethical questions related to this technique, as it is currently used in the evaluation of smoking prevention programs, also deserve careful consideration. Since legitimate techniques do exist to detect smoking behavior through the analysis of biological samples, some evaluators argue that the collection of such samples without the intent to analyze them is not "bogus" at all but simply a "pipeline." Others claim that this procedure does not deceive youth if the biological data are analyzed, even though technical limitations preclude using analytical results to draw conclusions. Those who advance such arguments perceive no need to debrief young people after the use of the bogus pipeline; indeed, they point out that such debriefing would hamper the technique's repeated use in longitudinal evaluations with multiple data collection points. The present author remains unconvinced of this need and troubled by the ethics of the bogus pipeline procedure.

Directions for Resolving Ethical and Methodological Issues

When self-reports of sensitive behaviors are critical to health program evaluation, the evaluator must attempt to resolve numerous methodological and ethical issues in developing the evaluation plan. The preceding discussion shows that these issues are intertwined and that important keys to unraveling them lie in respondents' motives for misreporting the performance of sensitive behaviors. The following directions for health program evaluation may prove fruitful.

Clear Definition of the Behavioral Information Needed. Although program objectives customarily define outcome indicators for evaluation, the behaviors that a program seeks to influence may be too loosely defined to guide plans for the collection of behavioral self-reports. Therefore, the evaluator should become familiar with the scientific evidence that links the targeted behaviors to health risks. As a further precaution, an epidemiologist should be asked to review draft questions, to ensure that the self-report data to be gathered will address the behavioral issues most critical to the health of the population studied.

Establishing the scientific relationship of sensitive behaviors to health status focuses the evaluation effort and provides a firm rationale for describing the purpose of data collection to others, including those who will be approached for personal information. Once this is done, the evaluator may find it useful to identify other behaviors prerequisite to the performance of the critical behaviors, both because questions on such corollary actions can lead up to the most sensitive items in data collection and because the information thus obtained can flag obstacles that future programs should explicitly address. Accordingly, questions to sexually active teenagers about their use of condoms during intercourse could be preceded by inquiries about their experiences in obtaining condoms and in negotiating condom use with a partner.

Early planning for data analysis will further indicate how detailed the data on individual behavior need to be. Requests for sensitive information can be limited to precoded response categories when plans indicate that behavioral data will be treated categorically or in terms of group statistics. A parsimonious approach to data collection is both ethically responsible and methodologically wise because, in minimizing invasion of respondents' privacy, the evaluator is likely to enhance cooperation. Conversely, the evaluator who collects more information about sensitive behavior than is required risks being regarded as less than efficient by the scientific community and as a voyeur by those to whom requests for data are made.

Enlistment of Help from Representatives of the Population to Be Studied. Since the sensitivity of behavior is a function of perceived social norms and situational contexts, the evaluator needs a window into the world of those who will be asked to provide sensitive behavioral information. Representatives of the population to be studied are uniquely qualified to help the evaluator develop and implement an evaluation plan.

Such representatives can make major contributions to the development of the evaluation plan by providing insights into how the target behavior is viewed and talked about in the local culture. They also can help the evaluator understand the contexts in which behavior occurs and the meanings it holds for members of the study population, thereby providing clues about the particular forms of response bias that are likely to operate during data collection. Similarly, representatives can reveal the potential consequences and benefits of providing information about sensitive behavior from the perspective of those who will be asked to contribute data.

As this diagnostic phase of planning progresses, representatives of the study population can assist with many specific tasks. They can propose ways to explain the evaluation study to potential respondents in terms relevant to their concerns and frames of reference, thus increasing the likelihood of cooperation and honest reporting. They can identify procedures to minimize the perceived risks of disclosing sensitive behavior, and they can suggest ways to increase the benefits of participation in evaluation. In addition, since the populations most at risk for a health problem often have their own "street language" for sensitive behaviors, representatives can recommend forms of question wording that ensure understanding and minimize embarrassment. They also can assist in crafting data collection methods that are attuned to the special needs and characteristics of those who will be questioned. As particular problems arise, they can elicit additional advice from key informants in the target population or organize focus groups for this purpose. Representatives also can help to pretest data collection instruments and procedures, and they can provide their own observations and frank feedback from others to improve evaluation plans as they develop.

Perhaps most important, as representatives help the evaluator learn more about the study population, they also will learn more about the program to be studied and the health problem to which it is directed. In addition, as the evaluator and representatives share their specialized knowledge, collaborate in problem solving, and demonstrate mutual concern for the study population, trust will be developed. Understanding and trust will then be reflected, not only in the evaluation design but also in communication with the respondent group. These are the qualities that most techniques for improving the validity of behavioral self-reports aim to achieve, and they are at the heart of procedures for protecting human subjects in research and evaluation.

Since the populations to which many health programs are targeted may have limited formal education and lifestyles foreign to the evaluation specialist, methods for working effectively with representatives of these populations will need to be developed. This may be the most demanding but also the most productive new direction for strengthening health program evaluations that depend on self-reports of sensitive behaviors. In confronting this challenge, evaluators have an opportunity to develop new approaches that advance both the science and the ethics of evaluation practice.

References

Block, G. "A Review of Validations of Dietary Assessment Methods." *American Journal of Epidemiology*, 1982, *115* (4), 492–505.

Bradburn, N. M., Sudman, S., and Associates. *Improving Interview Method and Questionnaire Design: Response Effects to Threatening Questions in Survey Research.* San Francisco: Jossey-Bass, 1979.

Carr, J. W., and Marascuilo, L. A. "Optimal Randomized Response Models and Methods for Hypothesis Testing." *Journal of Educational Statistics*, 1982, *7* (4), 295–310.

Evans, R. I., Hansen, W., and Mittelmark, M. "Increasing the Validity of Self-Reports of Smoking Behavior in Children." *Journal of Applied Psychology*, 1977, *62*, 521–523.

Gorden, R. L. *Interviewing: Strategy, Techniques, and Tactics.* Homewood, Ill.: Dorsey Press, 1969.

Jones, E. E., and Sigall, H. "The Bogus Pipeline: A New Paradigm for Measuring Affect and Attitude." *Psychological Bulletin*, 1971, *76*, 349–364.

Kinsey, A. C., Pomeroy, W. B., and Martin, C. E., *Sexual Behavior in the Human Male.* Philadelphia: Saunders, 1948.

Kinsey, A. C., Pomeroy, W. B., Martin, C. E., and Gebbhard, P. H. *Sexual Behavior in the Human Female.* Philadelphia: Saunders, 1953.

Kristiansen, C. M., and Harding, C. M. "The Social Desirability of Preventive Health Behavior." *Public Health Reports*, 1984, *99* (4), 384–388.

McDowell, I., and Newell, C. *Measuring Health: A Guide to Rating Scales and Questionnaires.* New York: Oxford University Press, 1987.

McKennell, A. C. "Bias in the Reported Incidence of Smoking by Children." *International Journal of Epidemiology*, 1980, *9* (2), 167–177.

McPhee, S. J., Richard, R. J., and Solkowitz, S. N. "Performance of Cancer Screening in a University General Internal Medicine Practice." *Journal of General Internal Medicine*, 1986, *1*, 275–281.

Midanik, L. "The Validity of Self-Reported Alcohol Consumption and Alcohol Problems: A Literature Review." *British Journal of Addiction*, 1982, *77*, 357–382.

Miller, P. V., and Groves, R. M. "Matching Survey Responses to Official Records: An Exploration of Validity in Victimization Reporting." *Public Opinion Quarterly*, 1985, *49*, 366–380.

Murray, D. M., and Perry, C. L. "The Measurement of Substance Use Among Adolescents: When Is the 'Bogus Pipeline' Method Needed?" *Addictive Behavior*, 1987, *12*, 225–233.

Phillips, B. S. *Social Research: Strategy and Tactics.* (2nd ed.) New York: Macmillan, 1971.

Rabow, J., and Neuman, C. A. "Garbaeology as a Method of Cross-Validating Interview Data on Sensitive Topics." *Sociology and Social Research*, 1984, *68* (4), 480–497.

Turner, C. F., and Martin, E. (eds.). *Surveying Subjective Phenomena.* Panel on Survey Measurement of Subjective Phenomena, Committee on National Statistics, Commission on Behavioral and Social Sciences and Education, National Research Council. 2 vols. New York: Russell Sage Foundation, 1984.

Turner, C. F., Miller, H. G., and Moses, L. E. (eds.). *AIDS: Sexual Behavior and Intravenous Drug Use.* Washington, D.C.: National Academy Press, 1989.

Warner, S. L. "Randomized Response: A Survey Technique for Eliminating Evasive Answer Bias." *Journal of the American Statistical Association,* 1965, *60,* 63–69.

Waterton, J. J., and Duffy, J. C. "A Comparison of Computer Interviewing Techniques and Traditional Methods in the Collection of Self-Report Alcohol Consumption Data in a Field Survey." *International Statistical Review,* 1984, *52* (2), 173–182.

Wyatt, G. E. "Reexamining Factors Predicting Afro-American and White American Women's Age of First Coitus." Unpublished paper, School of Medicine, University of California at Los Angeles, 1988.

Carol N. D'Onofrio is associate professor in the School of Public Health at the University of California, Berkeley. As principal investigator for large-scale studies on the prevention of adolescent tobacco use and as a consultant to numerous health agencies, she has been directly involved with ethical and methodological issues related to the use of behavioral self-reports in health program evaluations.

Considerations of purpose, feasibility, and statistical power,
as well as internal, external, and construct validity, determine
both the units of sample selection, randomization, treatment,
and observation and the analytical model one uses.

Levels of Analysis

David Koepke, Brian R. Flay

Many health promotion programs have several levels. For example, programs targeted at young people may feature school-based interventions, with sampling or treatment randomization at the school or classroom level. These programs produce hierarchical multilevel designs, having students within classes, within grade levels, within schools, within districts, and so forth. Other health promotion programs are also hierarchical, having patients of doctors within hospitals (or clinics), or employees within program groups within worksites, or members of families within communities. Assigning higher-level units (for example, schools, clinics, or communities) rather than individuals to treatment conditions adds another level to the hierarchy (such as students within schools within treatment conditions). This multilevel structure is often overlooked, sometimes with serious consequences. This chapter describes issues and approaches for the design and analysis of multilevel studies.

This paper uses the term *higher-level units* to refer to the entities (such as schools, clinics, worksites, or families) that consist of a collection of lower-level units (such as students, patients, employees, or family members). Other common terms for higher-level units apply only to specific statistical or application contexts: *clusters* (sampling), *blocks* (experimen-

This work was supported in part by the National Cancer Institute (CA34622, CA42760) and the National Institute on Drug Abuse (DA03468).

Marc T. Braverman (ed.). *Evaluating Health Promotion Programs.*
New Directions for Program Evaluation, no. 43. San Francisco: Jossey-Bass, Fall 1989.

tal design), *groups* or *aggregates* (social sciences), and *classes* (education). This chapter uses the term *individuals* to refer to the individual units at the lowest level of the hierarchy, which in most health promotion studies will be individual persons.

When using preexisting unit hierarchies, such as students in classes or patients in clinics or employees in worksites or members of families, one cannot consider the observations to be independent random samples of individuals. Rather, these are either (single-stage) cluster samples, if one uses every individual in each higher-level unit, or two-stage samples, if one samples only some individuals from each unit.

When one constructs new higher-level units (for example, smoking cessation or weight-loss groups) to deliver a program, the outcomes for members of these units will reflect unit-specific variation in the delivery of the treatment and other shared experiences. Outcomes may also reflect social influences of group members on one another's progress.

This lack of independence of observations for individuals within each higher-level unit, as well as considerations of internal, external, and construct validity, will have implications for study design and data analysis. These implications will affect choices of units of selection (which units to include in the study), assignment (which units at which level to randomize into different conditions), treatment (unit level at which to deliver intervention), observation (what unit characteristics to observe at each level), and analysis (how to model outcomes at each level by characteristics of the units at each level).

Nature of Study

The primary guide for design and analysis of a health promotion study is its purpose (Haney, 1980). Many studies assess the impact of an intervention compared to a control condition or compare effects of alternative interventions. In these instances, one can randomize treatment conditions by a unit other than the individual. Feasibility, cost, internal validity, external validity, construct validity, and statistical power to detect treatment effects all guide the choice of unit of randomization.

Other studies may examine an intervention applied to an entire school district or to an entire community without a control (for example, a pre-post design). In these cases, there is no assignment of units to conditions, but the sampling design remains an important issue. For evaluation of a school district, one could sample schools or classrooms for analysis, rather than individual students. For a community evaluation, one could sample residential blocks or households, rather than individual community members. Convenience, cost-effectiveness, the level at which the intervention is delivered, and the level at which it is designed to have its effect all guide the choice of sampling unit.

Other health promotion studies are correlational and only relate observed variables (health attitudes, beliefs, behavior of others) to health behaviors and outcomes. Even an evaluation of an intervention may have a correlational component that investigates process or covariates of health behaviors. Sampling may be by individuals or by higher-level units.

For any of these types of studies, one may have research questions about effects and/or variable relations at the individual level, at a higher level, or across levels. The remainder of this chapter focuses primarily on the first case, a randomized intervention study.

Sampling and Randomization

There are several reasons to sample by higher-level units or to randomize treatments by higher-level units instead of by individuals (Buck and Donner, 1982; Flay and Best, 1982). These concern feasibility, internal and external validity, construct validity, and statistical power.

Feasibility. It is convenient and usually more cost-effective to sample and to randomize treatment by higher-level units. There is a fixed cost per contact for data collection. A single interview can obtain health behavior information (smoking, current dieting, and so on) for an entire household. A single survey collection can obtain information from an entire classroom. A door-to-door survey of an entire residential block does not require the time and transit costs of a survey of geographically scattered, independently randomly sampled households. Even though data must be collected from a larger number of individuals to obtain equal statistical power, an equally statistically efficient cluster, or two-stage sample, is usually less expensive. Similarly, many health promotion programs deliver treatment to higher-level units (groups, classes, communities), rather than to individuals, by design. These treatments would be expensive to administer individually.

Beyond convenience, assignment to conditions at the individual level is not always possible. For example, it would be nearly impossible to limit exposure to communitywide promotions or mass media campaigns to specific individuals.

Internal Validity. Appropriate assignment by unit prevents or at least reduces contamination of conditions. By contrast, when one assigns members of preexisting groups to differing treatment conditions, subjects are likely to become aware of or even participate in the other conditions. Unit of assignment is not synonymous with unit of treatment, however. For example, one may assign entire schools to conditions to prevent contamination, although the health promotion is done at the classroom level.

Despite randomization, unit characteristics and intervention effects may be confounded (Flay and Cook, 1981). With only a few higher-level units per condition, the samples of units in different conditions are not likely to be comparable, and the study will effectively be reduced to a quasi-experiment. This is most easily illustrated by the trivial case in which only two units are assigned to two treatments. In this case, unit characteristics and treatment effects are inseparable. With a larger number of units, it is more likely that the samples of units randomly assigned to different conditions will be comparable. Deliberately stratifying units before randomization by variables that correlate with outcomes also may improve the assignment procedure.

External Validity. Many health promotion programs are provided within the setting of a higher-level unit, such as a school, community, or medical practice. One must determine the level of unit to which one wishes to make inferences from the results: to the behavior and health of individuals or to the community, school, medical practice, or other higher-level unit targeted. Selection and assignment by higher-level units is required for effectiveness trials, which assess how well an intervention or program works when delivered under real-world conditions (Flay, 1986). In general, one should sample at the level of unit to which one wishes to generalize the results. One should assign units to treatment at that level or higher.

One should also ensure that the units one selects reflect the range of units to which one wishes to generalize. When one independently randomly samples only a small number of higher-level units, the study may omit units of certain types (Flay and Cook, 1981). Again, one may use stratification—in this case, for selection of units—to ensure that the sample includes the full desired range of schools or clinics or communities, and so on.

Construct Validity. The level of observation should match the level at which a phenomenon occurs. It is difficult to infer effects and processes at one level from measures at another. Thus, if process within groups or classrooms is important, one should observe process directly at that level and not infer it from the responses of constituent individuals. Similarly, if individual outcomes are important, one should observe individuals and not infer individual outcomes from statistics on group outcomes.

Having too few units per condition can affect the construct validity of the treatment factor itself (Flay and Cook, 1981). Treatment may be confounded with the specific implementation, which depends on who delivers the program, relative stress on different program components, and local treatment definition.

Statistical Power. Observed outcomes for individuals within each higher-level unit are usually not independent. Because they are not independent, sampling by higher-level units is usually less efficient (in a statistical sense) than independent random sampling of individuals; that is, a study would require more individuals sampled by higher-level units than individuals independently randomly sampled to obtain the same precision of estimates and power for hypothesis testing (Cornfield, 1978).

The degree to which individuals within higher-level units have similar outcomes is measured by the *intraclass correlation,* the correlation between higher-level units and outcomes. The relative efficiency of the sampling design, or *design effect,* is the ratio of the number of individuals needed when complex sampling is used to the number needed when independent random sampling is used, to obtain equal statistical power. The design effect depends both on the intraclass correlation and on the number of individuals sampled from each higher-level unit. Specifically, for a large range of statistics for both cluster and two-stage sampling,

$$\text{equivalent number independently randomly sampled} = \frac{(\text{no. units}) \times (\text{no. per unit})}{\text{design effect}}$$

where design effect = 1 + (no. per unit − 1) × (intraclass correlation).

Thus, with eleven individuals per higher-level unit and an intraclass correlation for these units of .20, one needs to have three times as many individuals as if one independently randomly sampled individuals. The sampling-design effect increases quickly with number per higher-level unit. Therefore, it is usually more statistically efficient to collect small samples from a larger number of higher-level units (for example, schools or physicians' practices) than to collect exhaustive samples from a smaller number of these units. For example, with an intraclass correlation of .20, eleven units of size 21 (231 individuals) are equivalent to 46 individuals independently randomly sampled. This is more powerful than nine units of size 1,001 (9,090 individuals), which is equal to only 45 independently randomly sampled individuals. With even a moderate intraclass correlation, increasing the number of individuals sampled from each higher-level unit increases power very little (Hsieh, 1988).

Donner (1982) provides an excellent illustration of the effects of intraclass correlation and unit of selection (spouse pair, medical practice, or county) for four typical public health measures: hypertension, smoking, drinking, and body fat. Intraclass correlations for these measures at the family level range from .11 to .25 but only from .0026 to .0076 at the medical-practice level and from .0003 to .0071 at the county level. Nevertheless, because the number of individuals in each county is so large, design effects are much larger for county-level data (range 1.72 to 16.42) than for medical practices (1.47 to 6.28) or spouse pairs (1.11 to 1.25).

To determine power and required sample sizes, one therefore needs an estimate of the intraclass correlation, the number of units at each level available for sampling, and the typical number per higher-level unit. Several authors provide tables, formulas, or power curves to determine number of units and number per unit for desired power with specified effect size for continuous or binary outcomes (Barcikowski, 1981; Donner,

Birkett and Buck, 1981; Hsieh, 1988). Hsieh (1988) also includes power analyses for the case of stratified assignment of clusters.

Kish and Frankel (1974) noted that for many data sets the sampling-design effect for complex statistics such as regression coefficients tends to be much smaller than for simple statistics such as means, proportions, and differences between means or between proportions. Analytical results confirm this observation. Scott and Holt (1982) show that for two-stage samples the effective intraclass correlation for a regression is equal to the product of the intraclass correlation for the residuals and the intraclass correlation for the regressor. Thus, if each of these intraclass correlations were of moderate size, say, .20, the intraclass correlation for the regression estimates would be only .04. If each intraclass correlation were .005, the intraclass correlation for the regression estimate would be only .000025.

Nevertheless, the design effects for complex statistics can still be large enough to change the interpretation of statistical analyses. Lee, Forthofer, and Lorimor (1986) illustrate this with three examples from complex surveys: prevalence of mental disorders, length of hospital stays for psychiatric patients, and dietary patterns among the elderly. Predictors included demographics, type of hospital, and type of living arrangement. Standard errors for complex statistics such as regression coefficients and odds ratios, as well as hypothesis tests in analysis of variance (ANOVA) and contingency table analysis, were less affected than were standard errors for prevalence rates and means. However, several hypothesis tests were no longer "significant" once the sampling design was taken into consideration.

Landis, Lepkowski, Eklund, and Stehouwer (1982) obtained similar results with data from the first National Health and Nutrition Examination Survey. This complex survey sampled individuals within clusters of households within selected census districts. Multiple regression, analysis of variance, and chi-square contingency table tests were used to assess the effects of dietary habits (sweets and calories ingested), alcohol consumption, cigarette smoking, race, and sex on dental condition (periodontal index; sum of decayed, missing, and filled teeth) and Quetelet's body-mass index. The design effects for many of these complex statistics were greater than two, and some were greater than four—large enough to increase markedly the widths of confidence intervals.

Multilevel Data and Contextual Effects

Many analyses of health promotion programs focus on choosing an appropriate level or unit of analysis and determining whether a program has had an effect at that level. Such studies overlook the inherent multi-level nature of programs as well as of data and the possibility of inter-active or contextual effects.

The important task in analyzing multilevel data is the choice of analytical model, rather than unit of analysis (Burstein, 1980). There are many reasons to analyze data explicitly as multilevel. Important phenomena occur at all levels, effects at both the individual and higher level are important, it is difficult to make inferences across levels, and characteristics of different levels may interact.

Interactive effects may include differential responses of units to an intervention and differing relations among variables across units. Contextual effects are interactive effects of unit characteristics (including characteristics of other unit members and their outcomes) with individual characteristics on individual outcomes. Interactive and contextual effects have serious implications for the evaluation of health promotion programs and the design of further interventions. A program that affects only certain kinds of units or requires a synergy of individual and unit characteristics for greatest effect has implications different from those for a treatment that affects all individuals equally.

Multilevel models address these issues. A multilevel analysis simultaneously estimates the effects of predictors (including treatment condition) at each level on outcomes. These effects may include interactions of variables at different levels. For example, a multilevel analysis of a school-based health promotion program could assess the effects of school characteristics, health educator/program characteristics, baseline health beliefs of students, and their interactions on subsequent health behaviors of students.

Educational and sociological methodologists long have been concerned with issues of multilevel data and contextual effects (Blalock, 1984; Boyd and Iverson, 1979; Burstein, 1980; Firebaugh, 1980). By contrast, these issues are relatively unknown in the health promotion field.

Data Analysis

One can analyze data from a multilevel study in several ways. Most often, researchers simply analyze the data at a single level, using either data for individuals or data aggregated to higher-level units. Either choice presents difficulties. One alternative method treats a study as any other cluster or two-stage sample and uses methods developed for survey analysis to obtain estimates of statistics with appropriate standard errors and correct hypothesis tests (see Landis, Lepkowski, Eklund, and Stehouwer, 1982; Lee, Forthofer, and Lorimor, 1986). Another alternative method models the dependence of cases within clusters as a random effect (the mixed-model or variance component approach). Recently, several multilevel models and estimation methods have been developed that greatly extend the basic mixed-model/variance component approach.

Analysis at the Individual Level. One should not analyze individual-level data without regard to the sampling plan. This approach will underestimate the standard errors for statistics and grossly increase the Type I error rate for both continuous (Barcikowski, 1981; Blair, Higgins, Topping, and Mortimer, 1983) and categorical (Holt, Scott, and Ewings, 1980) data. Type I error rates (for a nominal .05 level) exceeding 50 percent are not uncommon for data analyzed incorrectly at the individual level.

Some researchers have made simple attempts to assess contextual effects in analyses at the individual level by including both higher-level unit means and individual-level values as predictors of individual-level outcomes (Boyd and Iverson, 1979). This introduces severe methodological difficulties (see Aitkin and Longford, 1986; Blalock, 1984; Burstein, 1980; Firebaugh, 1980). Aggregating individual-level information to a higher-unit level does not address the problem of statistical independence because the analysis remains at the individual level. Higher-level unit means and individual-level values are dependent. Thus, this approach is inadequate.

Analysis of Aggregate Data. One commonly recommended approach (for example, Barcikowski, 1981) is first to aggregate the outcome values for individuals within each higher-level unit (for example, obtain means or proportions) and then to analyze the aggregated data at that level. This is not without concerns (Roberts and Burstein, 1980). If one aggregates data to analyze at only the higher-unit level, one does overcome the problem of nonindependence that one would face at the individual level. From the results, one can properly make inferences at the aggregated-unit level. However, if one wishes to infer the effects of programs, or the relations of program variables to individual behaviors and outcomes, one must then deal with the considerable problems of cross-level or ecological inference (Glick, 1980; Morgenstern, 1982). It may not be possible to make inferences about the effects of health promotion programs on individuals. Further, it becomes impossible to assess individual differences or contextual effects. Because one cannot include individual-level factors and covariates, one loses the power increase and theoretical insight that one can realize with individual-level variables that explain portions of outcome variability.

Mixed or Variance-Component Models. One widely used approach to multilevel data treats differences among units at each level of the hierarchy (including the individual level) as random effects and differences due to treatments and other study factors as fixed effects (Goldstein, 1987; Hopkins, 1982). These models partition observed error variances into components that are due to each random factor. In a study of students within classes within schools, there would be separate "variance components" for students, for classes, and for schools. When the intraclass correlation is 0 for a particular level—that is, where units are entirely independent of the study outcome variables—the variance component for units at that level is also 0. In this case, the methods reduce to analysis at the individual level.

For continuous outcome variables and balanced data (equal numbers of observations per higher-level unit), one can apply these models using standard ANOVA methods (Hopkins, 1982). Consider a design having students within classes nested within treatment conditions. For this design, one would use the mean square for "class nested within treatment" as the error term for the treatment effect. In this balanced design case, the result for the treatment effect is identical to what one would obtain by analyzing aggregated data (class means). The mean square for "students within class" is the error term to test the class effect. If the class effect were not significant, one could use the pooled student and class effects as an error term, for a more powerful test of the treatment effect.

With unbalanced designs, the error terms for significance tests are more difficult to determine (Millikin and Johnson, 1984). For such models, one may use the general mixed model for continuous outcomes, as implemented in the BMDP 3V program.

The advantage of this mixed-model approach over analysis of aggregated data is that one can extend the model to include individual-level covariates and interaction effects of treatment with individual or higher-level unit characteristics. This approach is also applied in the context of regression analysis (Pfefferman and Smith, 1985; Rosner, 1984) and has been extended to binary outcomes as well (Anderson and Aitkin, 1985; Goldstein, 1987; Prentice, 1988).

Multilevel Analysis. Recently, several extensions of the mixed model to multilevel data, as well as algorithms to estimate these models, have been developed (DeLeeuw and Kreft, 1986; Goldstein, 1987; Longford, 1987; Mason, Wong and Entwisle, 1983; Raudenbush and Bryk, 1986).

The basic multilevel model is the hierarchical mixed-effects model presented in the preceding section. This model represents individual-level outcomes as a constant (intercept) term plus random effects for individuals and for higher-level units. To this basic model one can add both individual-level and higher-level unit predictors of individual-level outcomes. This assumes the same processes and equal effects for all higher-level units.

If treatment effects or processes were to differ across units, this would have strong evaluation implications. This possibility can be tested within the multilevel model framework. First, one can allow the relation of outcomes to individual-level variables to differ across units. In this case, each higher-level unit has its own regression-coefficient estimates for the regression of individual-level outcomes on individual-level predictors. If these regressions are found to differ across units, one then can add terms that relate higher-level unit variables to these within-unit coefficients. This procedure refines earlier "slopes as outcomes" methods (Burstein, 1980) and assesses the interaction of higher-level unit variables with individual-level variables.

Not all problems with multilevel analysis have been solved (see Bock, 1989; Raudenbush, 1988). Nevertheless, multilevel models have distinct advantages and are well enough developed to have many potential applications to the evaluation of health promotion programs. As more expository books (such as Bock, 1989; Goldstein, 1987) and accessible software become available, we expect to see widespread application of these models.

Recommendations

The preceding considerations suggest several specific conclusions and recommendations.

1. Sample at the lowest level at which one delivers an intervention or at which one expects unit effects.

2. Obtain an estimate of higher-level unit effects on outcome (the intraclass correlation) to estimate the number of units of desired size needed for required power.

3. Include several higher-level units per condition (if feasible) to decrease possible confounding of unit characteristics and treatment effects and to increase the range of units to which one can generalize results. When treatments are expensive, one can reduce costs by sampling more control units, which have only a data collection cost.

4. Add higher-level units to increase power, rather than increasing the number sampled per unit. Small samples from a larger number of higher-level units can have greater power than exhaustive samples from a smaller number of units.

5. Stratify units before selection, to guarantee that the sample includes every type of unit to which one wishes to generalize.

6. Stratify (block) units before randomized assignment by variables related to outcomes, to increase comparability of units across conditions and to increase the precision of effect estimates and power for hypothesis tests.

7. Do not analyze treatment effects at the individual level. Even a small intraclass correlation can result in a large design effect, with devastating effects on the validity of hypothesis tests. Type I error rates greater than 50 percent are not uncommon for tests of differences between conditions.

8. Regression analyses and other complex statistics have smaller design effects than do simple descriptive statistics. Nevertheless, one should employ some procedure that addresses the sampling plan, to avoid erroneous conclusions.

9. It is not necessary to aggregate data to obtain correct hypothesis tests. Mixed models provide the same results as does analysis of aggregated data while providing far greater flexibility. One cannot

infer individual-level relations from regression and other analyses on aggregated data.

10. Multilevel analyses allow one to study interactive and contextual effects that can have profound implications for health promotion.

References

Aitkin, M., and Longford, N. T. "Statistical Modeling Issues in School Effectiveness Studies (with Discussion)." *Journal of the Royal Statistical Society, Series A,* 1986, *149* (1), 1–43.

Anderson, D. A., and Aitkin, M. "Variance Component Models with Binary Response: Interviewer Variability." *Journal of the Royal Statistical Society, Series B,* 1985, *47* (2), 203–210.

Barcikowski, R. S. "Statistical Power with Group Means as the Unit of Analysis." *Journal of Educational Statistics,* 1981, *6* (3), 267–285.

Blair, R. C., Higgins, J. J., Topping, M. E., and Mortimer, A. L. "An Investigation of the Robustness of the *t* Test to Unit of Analysis Violations." *Educational and Psychological Measurement,* 1983, *43* (1), 69–80.

Blalock, H. M. "Contextual-Effects Models: Theoretical and Methodological Issues." *Annual Review of Sociology,* 1984, *10,* 353–372.

Bock, R. D. (ed.). *Multilevel Analysis of Educational Data.* Orlando, Fla.: Academic Press, 1989.

Boyd, L. H., and Iverson, G. R. *Contextual Analysis: Concepts and Statistical Techniques.* Belmont, Calif.: Wadsworth, 1979.

Buck, C., and Donner, A. "The Design of Controlled Experiments in the Evaluation of Non-Therapeutic Interventions." *Journal of Chronic Diseases,* 1982, *35,* 531–538.

Burstein, L. "The Analysis of Multilevel Data in Educational Research and Evaluation." In D. Berliner (ed.), *Review of Research in Education.* Vol. 8. Washington, D.C.: American Educational Research Association, 1980.

Cornfield, J. "Randomization by Group: A Formal Analysis." *American Journal of Epidemiology,* 1978, *108* (2), 100–102.

DeLeeuw, J., and Kreft, I. "Random Coefficient Models for Multilevel Analysis." *Journal of Educational Statistics,* 1986, *11* (1), 57–85.

Donner, A. "An Empirical Study of Cluster Randomization." *International Journal of Epidemiology,* 1982, *11* (3), 283–286.

Donner, A., Birkett, N., and Buck, C. "Randomization by Cluster: Sample-Size Requirements and Analysis." *American Journal of Epidemiology,* 1981, *114* (6), 906–914.

Firebaugh, G. "Groups as Contexts and Frog Ponds." In K. H. Roberts and L. Burstein (eds.), *Issues in Aggregation.* New Directions for Methodology of Social and Behavioral Science, no. 6. San Francisco: Jossey-Bass, 1980.

Flay, B. R. "Efficacy and Effectiveness Trials (and Other Phases of Research) in the Development of Health Promotion Programs." *Preventive Medicine,* 1986, *15,* 451–474.

Flay, B. R., and Best, J. A. "Overcoming Design Problems in Evaluating Health Behavior Programs." *Evaluation and the Health Professions,* 1982, *5* (1), 43–69.

Flay, B. R., and Cook, T. D. "Evaluation of Mass Media Prevention Campaigns." In R. E. Rice and W. J. Paisley (eds.), *Public Communications Campaigns.* Newbury Park, Calif.: Sage, 1981.

Glick, W. "Problems in Cross-Level Inferences." In K. H. Roberts and L. Burstein (eds.), *Issues in Aggregation*. New Directions for Methodology of Social and Behavioral Science, no. 6. San Francisco: Jossey-Bass, 1980.

Goldstein, H. *Multilevel Models in Educational and Social Research*. New York: Oxford University Press, 1987.

Haney, W. "Units and Levels of Analysis in Large-Scale Evaluation." In K. H. Roberts and L. Burstein (eds.), *Issues in Aggregation*. New Directions for Methodology of Social and Behavioral Science, no. 6. San Francisco: Jossey-Bass, 1980.

Holt, D., Scott, A. J., and Ewings, P. D. "Chi-Squared Tests with Survey Data." *Journal of the Royal Statistical Society, Series A*, 1980, *143*, 303-320.

Hopkins, K. D. "The Unit of Analysis: Group Means Versus Individual Observations." *American Educational Research Journal*, 1982, *19* (1), 5-18.

Hsieh, F. Y. "Sample Size Formulae for Intervention Studies with the Cluster as Unit of Randomization." *Statistics in Medicine*, 1988, *8*, 1195-1201.

Kish, L., and Frankel, M. "Inference from Complex Samples (with Discussion)." *Journal of the Royal Statistical Society, Series B*, 1974, *36*, 1-37.

Landis, J., Lepkowski, S., Eklund, S., and Stehouwer, S. "A Statistical Methodology for Analyzing Data from a Complex Survey, the First National Health and Nutrition Examination Survey." *Vital and Health Statistics, Series 2*, 92, DHHS Publication No. 82-1366. Washington, D.C.: U.S. Government Printing Office, 1982.

Lee, E. S., Forthofer, R. N., and Lorimor, R. J. "Analysis of Complex Sample Survey Data: Problems and Strategies." *Sociological Methods and Research*, 1986, *15* (1), 69-100.

Longford, N. T. "A Fast Scoring Algorithm for Maximum Likelihood Estimation in Unbalanced Mixed Models with Nested Random Effects." *Biometrika*, 1987, *74* (4), 817-827.

Mason, W. M., Wong, G. Y., and Entwisle, B. "Contextual Analysis Through the Multilevel Linear Model." In S. Leinhardt (ed.), *Sociological Methodology, 1983-1984*. San Francisco: Jossey-Bass, 1983.

Millikin, G. A., and Johnson, D. E. *Analysis of Messy Data*. Vol. 1. *Designed Experiments*. Belmont, Calif.: Wadsworth, 1984.

Morgenstern, H. "Uses of Ecological Analysis in Epidemiologic Research." *American Journal of Public Health*, 1982, 72 (12), 1336-1344.

Pfefferman, D., and Smith, T.M.F. "Regression Models for Grouped Populations in Cross-Section Surveys." *International Statistical Review*, 1985, *53* (1), 37-59.

Prentice, R. L. "Correlated Binary Regression with Covariates Specific to Each Binary Observation." *Biometrics*, 1988, *44*, 1033-1048.

Raudenbush, S. W. "Educational Applications of Hierarchical Linear Models: A Review." *Journal of Educational Statistics*, 1988, *13* (2), 85-116.

Raudenbush, S. W., and Bryk, A. S. "A Hierarchical Model for Studying School Effects." *Sociology of Education*, 1986, *59*, 1-17.

Roberts, K. H., and Burstein, L. (eds.). *Issues in Aggregation*. New Directions for Methodology of Social and Behavioral Science, no. 6. San Francisco: Jossey-Bass, 1980.

Rosner, B. "Multivariate Methods in Ophthalmology with Application to Other Paired Data Situations." *Biometrics*, 1984, *40*, 1025-1035.

Scott, A. J., and Holt, D. "The Effect of Two-Stage Sampling on Ordinary Least-Squares Methods." *Journal of the American Statistical Association*, 1982, 77, 848-854.

David Koepke is associate director for statistical research, Prevention Research Center, School of Public Health, University of Illinois at Chicago.

Brian R. Flay is associate professor of public health and director of the Prevention Research Center, School of Public Health, University of Illinois at Chicago.

*Difficulties in identifying no-treatment baselines for
comparison with media effects in health promotion
programming are caused by the self-selective nature of media
exposure and a reliance on nonequivalent comparison groups.
Two potential evaluation design solutions that avoid these
problems are presented and discussed.*

Evaluation of Health Promotion Media Campaigns

Jack McKillip

A consistent and central component of health promotion interventions is the use of media, such as newspapers and television, to educate about a health behavior and to provide training in its adoption or extinction (see, for example, Greenberg and Gantz, 1976; Jason and others, 1988; McKillip, Landis, and Phillips, 1984). Despite a rich history and wide popularity, unique aspects of mass media contribute to the absence of clear evidence of their utility (McGuire, 1986). A chief cause of the ambiguous assessment of media effects is the difficulty of identifying no-treatment baselines for comparison with measurements of media effects (Flay and Cook, 1981).

Two aspects of mass media that complicate evaluation are self-selection of exposure and availability of media to entire groups. Since most people have a choice of which media messages they will be exposed to, viewing and processing these messages results from an interaction between the media stimulus and characteristics of audience members. Simple comparisons of those who saw a message with those who did not can confound differences in exposure to health media with differences in interest and knowledge of a topic, in motivation to change, and in need for information on the topic.

While actual audiences often differ from potential audiences, people

Marc T. Braverman (ed.). *Evaluating Health Promotion Programs.*
New Directions for Program Evaluation, no. 43. San Francisco: Jossey-Bass, Fall 1989.

who are not in the potential audience often come from different populations than those who are (*population* is used here in a statistical and not necessarily a demographic sense). Television, radio, newspapers, and even billboards and bus posters are available across wide geographical areas. Nonexposed groups must come from some place other than the location of the (potentially) exposed group. Even when the logistical problems associated with finding and measuring distant populations are surmounted, the multiple preexisting differences between the exposed and the nonexposed groups obscure the inference that observed postmedia differences are due to media programming.

Evaluation Designs Used with Health Promotion Media Campaigns

Difficulties in identifying no-treatment baselines for comparison with media effects in health promotion programming have led evaluators down a number of different paths. Some of these are useful for evaluating media effects, and others address quite different questions. Four approaches will be reviewed briefly in order to illuminate the general problem.

Studying the Actual Audience. In this case, only that part of the potential audience that is actually reached by the health promotion media campaign is interviewed. Measurements include data on characteristics and experiences that are relevant for identifying media exposure and impact. Often an audience-initiated contact is used to identify respondents for later interview by the evaluators. For example, Best (1980) studied a six-session smoking modification television campaign. Respondents were selected from among viewers who requested a self-help guide developed to accompany the program. Using mail and telephone follow-ups, evaluators were able to identify light and heavy users of the promotional media and materials. The heavy-versus-light user dichotomy was related to respondents' characteristics and to self-reported impact on smoking behavior. Even the finding that heavy users showed greater impact than light users would not indicate that the media campaign was the cause of this difference, since the dichotomy was correlated with a number of factors besides exposure. Comparison of impact on those surveyed with normative information about other smoking modification approaches is similarly confounded.

Comparing the Actual Audience with Those Not Exposed to the Media Message. In this case, a probability sample of the potential audience is interviewed. Respondents are dichotomized into those reporting exposure to the health promotion message and those reporting no exsure. The two groups can be compared on individual characteristics, as well as on program-related knowledge, attitudes, and behaviors. For example, Greenberg and Gantz (1976) studied an hour-long TV program aimed at affecting knowledge and beliefs about sexually transmitted diseases (STDs). Telephone interviews were conducted with a large sample of the potential audience after one of several screenings of the program. Program viewers were found to be more knowledgeable about STDs than nonviewers were. Whether this difference was due to exposure to the program, to factors that led to exposure, or to the interaction of these variables is not clear.

Interpretation of comparisons between exposed and nonexposed members of a potential audience, as between heavy and light media users, is complicated by what Cook and Campbell (1979) label a "selection" artifact: Preexisting differences between groups may account for effects that might otherwise be attributed to media programming.

Comparing Media-Augmented Programming with Media-Only Controls. In this case, a probability sample of the potential audience is selected for observation before and after the health promotion media programming. Rather than being divided according to self-selected exposure, groups are created through random selection of part of the sample to receive a nonmedia intervention aimed at strengthening the impact of the media programming. Changes from pre- to post-observations of knowledge, attitudes, and behavior are compared for the two groups.

A recent example is provided by Jason and others' (1988) study of a TV news–based smoking modification intervention. Twice every weekday for four weeks, the news broadcast of a large, urban, independent TV station carried parts of a smoking modification program. In addition, the media programming was augmented by a manual, distributed widely within the area served by the TV station. A mostly minority sample of smokers in the potential audience was interviewed before and after the media intervention. Respondents were randomly divided into two groups: An experimental group that was mailed the program manual, received phone encouragement to participate, and was offered neighborhood group support meetings; and a comparison group that had the TV programming and manual available only as members of the potential audience. Even though there were observed postobservation differences in smoking, the role of the TV campaign is not clear. The experimental group differed from the comparison group because of the support and encouragement intervention as well as reported exposure to the media message. Support and encouragement, alone or in interaction with the measurement procedures, might have produced the smoking impact without the TV campaign (compare Cook and others, 1982).

Using a Comparison Population from a Different Geographical Area. In this case, pre- and postobservations on members of the potential media audience are compared with observations on a comparable sample living outside the reach of the health promotion campaign, thus avoiding selection problems confounded with nonexposure among potential audience members. Perhaps the most famous recent example of this design is the Stanford Three Communities Project (Farquhar and others, 1977). Respondents from two towns that shared media outlets were compared to those from a third town, which because of distance and other factors was served by different outlets. Extensive media programming about risk factors for cardiovascular disease was carried out over a two-year period. In addition, a sample of respondents in one of the experimental towns was selected for an intensive support intervention. Effects attributable to media interventions were found for knowledge and self-reported change in diet.

By comparing members of the potential media audience with a group from a different geographical area, the design of the project avoided the selection problems already discussed. However, interpretation of impacts was obscured by other factors related to use of a "control town." First, historical events (other than the intervention) localized in a single town may have influenced health behaviors, especially in the less closely monitored control town. Second, Type I errors due to violation of independence assumptions may have led to overidentification of effects, since residents of a single town share many sources of variance in addition to the "independent variables" (Leventhal, Safr, Cleary, and Gutmann, 1980; Koepke and Flay, this volume). Third, interaction of measurement procedures with media programming may have produced an effect. This latter issue is especially relevant for media evaluations that use an agenda-setting approach (Roberts and Maccoby, 1985). In the Stanford project (Farquhar and others, 1977), measurement included four eighty-minute sessions for each respondent. This measurement process was probably extremely reactive. Earlier measures may have affected later measures or interacted with media programming to affect later measurement. For example, while there is apparently little empirical evidence that political media messages affect voting behavior, answering questions about voting does (McGuire, 1986).

Alternative Evaluation Designs

The approaches just reviewed are problematic for the evaluation of health promotion media effects. They do not address the question of media impact directly. Because of potential selection artifacts, they do not provide unambiguous no-treatment baselines for comparisons with media effects. Moreover, reactivity of repeated measurement may sensitize parts of the audience to media programming and thus become a de facto part of the intervention itself. In addition, the use of a comparison group to generate a no-treatment baseline increases logistical and financial burdens for the evaluation: Observations need to be taken on both the targeted and the comparison groups. The expense of evaluation is particularly acute when programming has a narrow geographical focus or is not part of a major research project. The following two evaluation designs have potential for providing relatively unambiguous information on media impacts while requiring only that data be gathered from a single population.

Multiple Baselines Across Behaviors. A multiple-baselines-across-behaviors (MBAB) design is a single-case experimental design used in animal laboratory research or in treatment and management situations where evaluation is routine and emphasis is on producing changes in relatively few individuals (Barlow and Hersen, 1984; Kazdin and Tuma, 1982). It combines multiple observations, multiple measures, abrupt onset of interventions, and replication to produce internally valid evidence of intervention impact. An MBAB design has the following characteristics:

1. Multiple, independent behaviors are observed for a single subject (or other observation unit) during the entire study.
2. After relatively stable observed baselines are established, an intervention is abruptly introduced to produce changes on one of the baseline measures. If this targeted measure changes when the intervention is introduced and the other measures remain stable, support is provided for the impact of the intervention. (Statistical analyses are possible but not typical.)
3. A second intervention is abruptly introduced to produce changes on another of the baseline measures. If this target measure changes when the intervention is introduced and the other measures remain stable, further support is provided for the impact of the intervention.
4. This pattern can be continued until interventions are introduced for all measures.

When applied outside the laboratory, single-case designs treat large groups as a single unit—for example, police patrol zones (Schnelle and others, 1977) or schools (Roberts, Fanurik, and Wilson, 1988). In evaluation of health promotion media campaigns, the "single subject" is the potential audience whose behavior is sampled by observing different audience samples at regular intervals over the course of study. Baseline "behaviors" can include knowledge of various health topics for which media programming will later be introduced. A pattern of changes in targeted health topic behaviors, coincident with the onset of media programming, indicates media impact.

McKillip, Lockhart, Eckert, and Phillips (1985) used an MBAB design as part of the evaluation of a media campaign aimed at encouraging responsible alcohol use by college students. Each week for a period of ten weeks, a different random sample of the student body was interviewed concerning two responsible-alcohol-use themes: "It is not rude to refuse a drink" and "Friends do not let friends drive drunk." After a two-week baseline period, a campuswide multimedia campaign on the first theme was introduced for two weeks. It included newspaper ads and articles, radio programming, and widespread placement of campaign posters. After another baseline period during the fourth and fifth weeks of the study, a two-week campaign was introduced on the second theme. Measurement continued for two weeks after media programming on the second theme had ended. Dependent measures were recall of media messages related to the two campaign themes.

Figure 1 presents results from the McKillip, Lockhart, Eckert, and Phillips (1985) study, illustrating the MBAB design. Recall of newspaper and poster messages showed discontinuity from precampaign baseline levels only at the outset of the specific campaigns. Effects were duplicated for both media and are replicated for both campaign themes. Note that recall of media related to the second campaign theme did not change during the campaign period concerning the first theme. While this study focused only on message recall, self-reported attitudes and behaviors related to the campaign themes can serve as baselines in the same manner as recall does in Figure 1.

In the MBAB design, observations on nontargeted measures provide no-treatment baselines for comparison with measures of media effects. Use of random samples from the same population for interviews or observations avoids testing and selection problems that affect other evaluation designs. Use of a single study population also cuts down on the logistical and financial burdens. Finally, the potential for replication of impact baseline measures makes the MBAB design stronger than many comparison-group designs for evaluation of media impacts.

Control Construct. One drawback of the MBAB design is that it requires phased introduction of multiple interventions. However, with a control construct design (similar to what Cook and Campbell, 1979, call a "non-equivalent dependent variable" design), the multiple-measures aspect of the MBAB design can be applied with a single intervention. The design uses two types of constructs. The experimental construct is a health issue that is the focus of a media intervention. It is represented by measures of knowledge, attitude, or behavior related to the targeted issue. Control constructs are health issues, similar to the experimental issue, for which no media intervention is planned. Control constructs are also represented by measures of knowledge, attitude, or behavior. Rather than estimating no-treatment baselines from groups not exposed to media, this design uses measures of constructs that are not the focus of media interventions. A control construct design has the following characteristics:

1. Multiple constructs are observed during the entire length of the study, including measures related to the media programming (experimental construct) and measures of similar constructs that could but will not be the focus of media intervention (control constructs).

Figure 1. Recall of Poster and Newspaper Ads Containing Campaign Themes

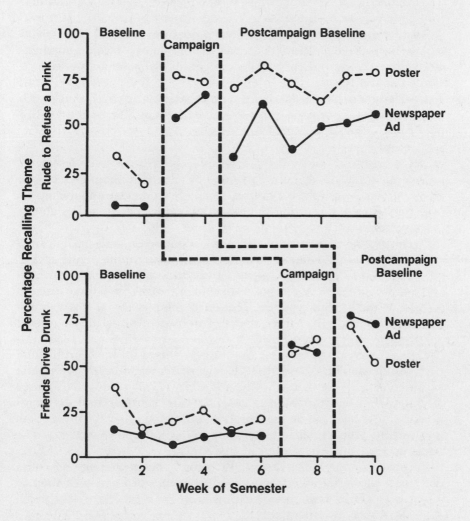

2. Measurements are taken at regular intervals before, during, and after the media programming, with a different sample of the study population measured at each observation time. Different samples are used in order to minimize the reactivity of measurement.

3. Media programming is introduced, usually abruptly, in a way that allows modeling of potential impact.

4. The specific form of the Construct × Time of Observation interaction expected for a single replication of the control construct
   design is tested in an analysis of variance (ANOVA) or similar
   statistical analysis format.

These steps can be illustrated by the procedures followed in Baldwin
and McKillip's (1989) control construct evaluation of a media campaign
aimed at increasing awareness of the dangers of STDs among students at
a large state university:

1. Measures of knowledge, belief, and behavior were collected relevant
   to the experimental construct—the dangers of STDs—and to two
   control constructs: moderate alcohol consumption and regular
   exercise.
2. On eight consecutive Thursday nights, a different random sample
   of the student body was interviewed by telephone about each of the
   constructs, with these measures: recall of media related to the topic,
   frequency of discussing the topic, and adherence to beliefs about
   the topic.
3. During the fifth week of the study, a one-week multimedia campaign on STD awareness was launched, using radio, newspapers,
   posters, and other promotions. It was expected that the campaign
   would have a strong initial impact on message recall, topic discussion, and belief acceptance. This effect was expected to decay gradually over the final three weeks of measurement, when no media
   programming was planned.

Figure 2 presents an example of results predicted for the control construct design, similar to those indicated by preliminary analyses for recall
and discussion in the Baldwin and McKillip (1989) study. The figure
illustrates little change on measures of the control construct, but a change
in trend line is observed on the measure of the experimental construct at
the time of the media campaign. The strong initial impact of the media
campaign gradually decreases in intensity.

In contrast to the MBAB design, the control construct design depends
on a single media intervention to present evidence of impact. In such a
case, it is especially important that powerful statistical analyses be used
to test the impact hypothesis.

In an ANOVA for a control construct design, media impact is revealed
as part of an interaction between a Constructs factor and a Time of
Observation factor. In the example of Figure 2, Constructs is a within-
subjects factor with two degrees of freedom (one experimental construct
and two control constructs). Time of Observation is a between-subjects
factor with seven degrees of freedom (the eight study weeks). The total
interaction has fourteen degrees of freedom and does not provide a sensitive test of the specific interaction effect hypothesized: an increase in the
experimental construct measure's trend line in week five that gradually

Figure 2. Sample Results for Control Construct Design

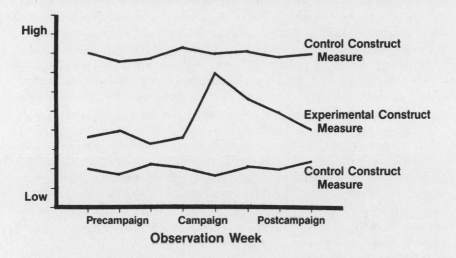

Note: There were one experimental and two control constructs and eight observation weeks. A one-week media campaign was introduced in the fifth observational week.

lessens, with no change in the two control construct measures' trend lines. A powerful test of a specific interaction is provided by contrast coding (for example, see Winer, 1971). This procedure is available as an option in most statistical analysis packages.

Contrasts, which each have one degree of freedom, are constructed by weighting main effects (Construct and Time of Measurement) to derive weights for interaction-cell values. In the present example, the experimental construct measure is contrasted with the control construct measures by giving the former a weight of 2 and each of the latter a weight of –1. The specific form of the media impact hypothesized would be captured using these weights with the Time of Observation factor: –3, –3, –3, –3, 6, 3, 2, 1. This contrast takes the form of a stable baseline, a positive impact of media programming on observation 5, and a gradual decline of this positive impact. The exact weights chosen are arbitrary but should sum to 0 and should reflect the pattern of impact hypothesized. The test of the hypothesis of media impact for the control construct design is provided by weighting the Constructs × Time of Observation interaction-cell values by both main-effects weights; the weight for each individual cell is determined by the product of the marginal cell weights. For example, the weight for the experimental construct measure during week 5 is 2 × 6 = 12. The resulting interaction contrast is tested against the normal interaction error term.

In the control construct design, the control constructs serve much the same function as control groups in the nonequivalent control group design (Cook and Campbell, 1979). A good control construct is like a good control group: It is similar to the experimental construct in terms of historical interest, social desirability, and measurement reliability. If carefully chosen, control constructs can help rule out such threats to internal validity as history, maturation, and instrumentation. Because the design observes respondents only once and selects respondents randomly from the same population, threats of selection and testing are not plausible.

Note on Appropriate Outcome Measures. Many variables have been used in studies of media impact, including self-reports of recall of media, attitudes and beliefs about health behaviors, health behaviors themselves, and physiological indicators related to health behavior. There is disagreement in the literature about the appropriate level of analysis. This disagreement reflects diversity in theoretical models of potential media impact (Nimmo and Sanders, 1981), as well as a penchant for a summative (for example, McGuire, 1986) rather than a causal-process (for example, Roberts and Maccoby, 1985) approach to evaluation. Use of either the MBAB design or the control construct design is consistent with most models of media impact and with either a summative or a causal-process approach to evaluation.

Summary

Both the MBAB and the control construct designs offer considerable logistical economies over comparison group designs because they involve only within-group comparisons. In addition, the designs provide the potential for valid inferences of health promotion media impacts, using replications and within-group comparisons to overcome internal validity threats afflicting the more traditional between-group designs. However, neither the MBAB nor the control construct design solves all evaluation problems for health media programming. Observation by random sampling from a population may not be sensitive to important effects, especially if the media campaign reaches only a small portion of a population. Media effects may not be replicated over health topics or themes. Control constructs may not be similar to experimental constructs on important factors, leading to increased or decreased sensitivity to media impacts. However, since the two designs reviewed here fit the typical media constraints of self-selected exposure and potential exposure of an entire population, and since they permit relatively clear no-treatment baselines, they will be useful in evaluating media effects where other designs are impractical or ambiguous.

Alone, the MBAB and control construct designs are probably most persuasive where the analogy between a single subject and the study population is strong—where the target population is relatively homogeneous in personal characteristics and in media use. The control construct design is compatible with and will considerably strengthen clarity of inferences from most traditional comparison group designs. The addition of measures for one or more control constructs will increase the cost of an evaluation much less than the addition of a nontreated comparison group.

References

Baldwin, K., and McKillip, J. *STDs in the 80s: The Evaluation of a Program to Increase Students' Awareness of the Dangers of Sexually Transmitted Diseases and the Effectiveness of Condoms at Preventing STDs.* Carbondale: Department of Psychology, Southern Illinois University, 1989.

Barlow, D. H., and Hersen, M. *Single-Case Experimental Designs.* (2nd ed.) Elmsford, N.Y.: Pergamon Press, 1984.

Best, J. A. "Mass Media, Self Management and Smoking Modification." In P. O. Davidson and S. M. Davidson (eds.), *Behavioral Medicine: Changing Health Lifestyles.* New York: Brunner, 1980.

Cook, T. D., Appleton, H., Conner, R. F., Shaffer, A., Tamkin, G., and Webster, S. J. *"Sesame Street" Revisited.* New York: Russell Sage Foundation, 1982.

Cook, T. D., and Campbell, D. T. *Quasi-Experimentation: Design and Analysis Issues for Field Settings.* Skokie, Ill: Rand McNally, 1979.

Farquhar, J. W., Maccoby, N., Wood, P. D., Alexander, J. K., Breitrose, H., Brown, B. W., Haskell, W. L., McAlister, A. L., Meyer, A. J., Nash, J. D., and Stern, M. P. "Community Education for Cardiovascular Health." *Lancet,* 1977, *4,* 1192–1195.

Flay, B. R., and Cook, T. D. "Evaluation of Mass Media Prevention Campaigns." In R. E. Rice and W. J. Paisley (eds.), *Public Communication Campaigns.* Newbury Park, Calif.: Sage, 1981.

Greenberg, B. S., and Gantz, W. "Public TV and Taboo Topics: The Impact of VD Blues." *Public Telecommunication Review,* 1976, *4,* 56–59.

Jason, L. A., Tait, E., Goodwin, D., Buckenberger, L., and Gruder, C. L. "Effects of a Televised Smoking Cessation Intervention Among Low-Income and Minority Smokers." *American Journal of Community Psychology,* 1988, *16,* 863–876.

Kazdin, A. E., and Tuma, A. H. (eds.). *Single-Case Research Designs.* New Directions for Methodology of Social and Behavioral Science, no. 13. San Francisco: Jossey-Bass, 1982.

Leventhal, H., Safr, M. A., Cleary, P. D., and Gutmann, M. "Cardiovascular Risk Modification by Community-Based Programs for Life Style Change: Comments on the Stanford Study." *Journal of Consulting and Clinical Psychology,* 1980, *48,* 150–158.

McGuire, W. J. "The Myth of Massive Media Impact: Savagings and Salvagings." In G. Comstock (ed.), *Public Communication Behavior.* Orlando, Fla.: Academic Press, 1986.

McKillip, J., Landis, S. M., and Phillips, J. "The Role of Advertising in Birth Control Use and Sexual Decision Making." *Journal of Sex Education and Therapy,* 1984, *10,* 44–48.

McKillip, J., Lockhart, D. C., Eckert, P. S., and Phillips, J. "Evaluation of a Responsible Alcohol Use Media Campaign on a College Campus." *Journal of Alcohol and Drug Education,* 1985, *30,* 88–97.

Nimmo, D. D., and Sanders, K. R. *Handbook of Political Communication.* Newbury Park, Calif: Sage, 1981.

Roberts, D. F., and Maccoby, N. "Effects of Mass Communication." In G. Lindzey and E. Aronson (eds.), *Handbook of Social Psychology,* Vol. 2. New York: Random House, 1985.

Roberts, M. C., Fanurik, D., and Wilson, D. R. "A Community Program to Reward Children's Use of Seat Belts." *American Journal of Community Psychology,* 1988, *16,* 395–407.

Schnelle, J. F., Kirchner, R. E., Casey, J. D., Uselton, P. H., and McNees, M. P. "Patrol Evaluation Research: A Multiple-Baseline Analysis of Saturation Police Patrolling During Day and Night Hours." *Journal of Applied Behavioral Analysis,* 1977, *10,* 33–40.

Winer, B. J. *Statistical Principles in Experimental Design.* New York: McGraw-Hill, 1971.

Jack McKillip is a professor of psychology at Southern Illinois University, Carbondale. He is coauthor of Decision Analysis for Program Evaluators *(Sage, 1984) and is the author of* Need Analysis: Tools for the Human Services and Education *(Sage, 1987).*

Preliminary guidelines are proposed to enhance the interpretability of outcomes in health promotion and disease prevention program evaluations.

Preliminary Guidelines for Reporting Outcome Evaluation Studies of Health Promotion and Disease Prevention Programs

Joel M. Moskowitz

In the past few decades, numerous primary prevention programs have been developed in an attempt to promote health or prevent disease. The target behaviors for these programs have typically included alcohol, tobacco and other drug use, sexual practices, diet, and exercise. Several hundred outcome (or summative) evaluations have been conducted to assess the effectiveness of these health promotion or disease prevention programs. Although most of these studies have employed experimental or quasi-experimental designs, reviews of this research commonly report that the conclusions drawn by many of these studies are unwarranted (Bruvold and Rundall, 1988; Flay, 1985; Moskowitz, 1989; Rothman and Byrne, 1981; Schaps and others, 1981). Problems that undermine the interpretability of this research include inappropriate comparison groups, sizable attrition rates, and inadequate measurement procedures and statistical analyses. Although such problems suggest to the careful reader

Marc T. Braverman (ed.). *Evaluating Health Promotion Programs.*
New Directions for Program Evaluation, no. 43. San Francisco: Jossey-Bass, Fall 1989.

alternative explanations for the findings, the evaluation reports often fail to discuss these explanations, or they dismiss them prematurely.

Health promotion and disease prevention evaluation studies have improved somewhat in recent years. For example, recent antismoking education studies are more likely to employ stronger designs than their earlier counterparts (Flay, 1985). However, many of these studies still suffer from problems with noncomparability of control groups and substantial subject attrition. Whereas most studies would benefit from supplementary statistical analyses aimed at ruling out rival hypotheses, it is rare to find such a sophisticated presentation of the data. Even in those studies where major methodological problems are not apparent, the documentation of methods and results is often inadequate for substantiating the findings because major details about the research have been omitted (Moskowitz, 1989). Thus, in part, the failure of outcome evaluations to provide results that merit the reader's confidence is due to inadequate documentation of methods and results, as well as to inadequate analysis of the data.

The interpretability of outcomes in health promotion and disease prevention evaluations would be substantially enhanced if researchers were to adopt existing standards. Based on input from more than a dozen professional organizations, two sets of general standards have been developed for conducting evaluation studies (ERS Standards Committee [ERSSC], 1982; Joint Committee on Standards for Educational Evaluation, 1981). In order to facilitate the adoption of these standards, it may be important to customize these standards for specific types of research. One field where this has occurred is in medical research that utilizes controlled clinical trials (Chalmers and others, 1981; Mosteller, Gilbert, and McPeek, 1980).

This chapter proposes preliminary guidelines for reporting health promotion and disease prevention program evaluations that employ pretest-posttest comparison group designs. Such guidelines should be useful for designing outcome evaluation studies, as well as for reporting and reviewing this research. The guidelines have been based on the ERS standards because these standards focus more specific attention on issues that affect the interpretability of results than do the Joint Committee Standards.

Because replicability is the sine qua non of scientific research, the authors of a socially significant evaluation study should assume that others will replicate it (Riecken and Boruch, 1974). Unfortunately, in the social sciences such replication is rare; thus, it is all the more important that the details of a study be adequately documented to enable critical reading. Otherwise, building a scientifically based literature through integrating the results of individual studies may be problematic. Until professional journals are willing to devote sufficient space for adequate reporting of evaluation studies, it is imperative that detailed technical reports be written to supplement any published papers about evaluation studies.

Evaluation Overview

The evaluation report should present both the *program theory,* the model that articulates how the program is supposed to work, and the *implementation process theory,* the model that describes the mechanism by which the program is delivered (Bickman, 1987). The structure and content of the program as designed should be described, and information should be provided about the scope and sequence of any curriculum used. The qualifications and training of the program-delivery agents, as well as any materials used in the training, should also be described.

If the comparison groups received any special interventions—for example, if there was a placebo control group—these interventions should also be described. Likewise, it is useful to describe what activities, if any, the program supplanted in the experimental condition.

Process Evaluation

The process evaluation describes the program as implemented, which is important for interpreting the results of an outcome evaluation. When an intervention is found to be effective, such data are essential to program dissemination, for it is necessary to understand how a program can deviate from its ideal and still meet its basic objectives (Patton, 1979). When an intervention is found to be ineffective or harmful to program participants, such data can help inform whether these outcomes are attributable to inadequate program implementation, design, or theory (Boruch and Gomez, 1979; Judd and Kenny, 1981).

The process evaluation should address how the program was implemented, including "what services were provided, to whom, when, how often, and in what settings" (Office for Substance Abuse Prevention, 1989, p. 7). In order to replicate the study or disseminate the program, it is useful to document systematically the nature and extent of any deviations from the program design. The process data may be used to determine the extent to which the program was delivered as designed—that is, to assess the fidelity of program implementation, or the extent to which the program was adapted, and whether the adaptations were conducive to program efficacy or were counterproductive (Bickman, 1987). Process data are also invaluable in revising a program and may provide insight into whether the program-delivery system needs alteration. The process data may be qualitative as well as quantitative and may consist of live observations or audio- and videotapes of program training and program delivery, feedback from program-delivery agents and participants via questionnaires or interviews, and records of participants' attendance or exposure to the program.

Research Design and Statistical Analysis

Subjects and Sampling. The demographic and socioeconomic characteristics of the target population should be reported, as well as any other factors that may influence the study's generalizability. In addition, any procedures employed to obtain the informed consent of subjects should be summarized.

According to the ERS Standards Committee (1982, p. 13), "if sampling is to be used, the details of the sampling methodology (choice of unit, method of selection, time frame, and so forth) should be described and justified, based on explicit analysis of the requirements of the evaluation, including generalization." Even if the study does not involve a probability sample, where every subject has a known probability of being selected, the factors that determined what subjects were included in the study must be provided. If social institutions (for example, schools) were recruited, then the criteria for their inclusion should be provided, as well as the rate of institutional participation. The number of subjects and participation rates at pretest should be presented for each experimental condition. The participation rates should be based on the number of subjects who were eligible for the study—that is, the number of subjects whom the researcher attempted to recruit, or the number enrolled in the participating institutions at the time of the pretest. The rates should be summarized for each of the major sources of nonparticipation, such as lack of subject consent, lack of parental consent (if applicable), or absence at pretest.

Outcome Measurement. "Justification should be provided that appropriate procedures and instruments have been specified. . . . The data collection and preparation procedures should provide safeguards so that the findings and reports are not distorted by any biases of data collectors" (ERS Standards Committee, 1982, pp. 13-14). The instruments should assess variables that are expected to be influenced by the intervention and that are appropriate to the age and composition of the sample. Sufficient detail should be provided about data collection procedures to enable replication. Generally, it is informative to present the results on all measures collected in the study. If this is not done, then appropriate justifications should be provided.

"The measurement methods and instruments should be specified and described, and their reliability and validity should be estimated for the population or phenomena to be measured. . . . The estimated validity and reliability of data collection instruments and procedures should be verified under the prevailing circumstances of their use" (ERS Standards

Committee, 1982, pp. 13–14). If possible, test-retest reliabilities should be presented for the sample, as well as internal consistency reliability estimates.

Information should be provided about the validity of the measures. It is often difficult, however, to validate health-compromising behaviors in a population where the prevalence and recency of such behaviors is low. Where biological measures are available, there are often problems with their sensitivity (that is, they can detect only very recent or extreme behavior) or with their specificity (that is, they detect behaviors other than the behavior of interest). Because of these limitations, multiple measures possessing complementary properties may be necessary. For example, in assessing cigarette smoking, one can analyze saliva samples for both thiocyanate, a sensitive but not very specific measure, and for cotinine, a specific but not very sensitive measure. Some studies report that relationships between biological and self-report measures are statistically significant but fail to report the more critical information about the magnitude of these relationships. This only indicates that the relationships are greater than zero. If the prevalence of recent behavior is low, then the magnitude of the relationships between the biological and the self-report measures may be too small to be meaningful for validation purposes. Thus, most studies must rely predominantly on subjects' self-reports about the outcomes of interest.

Self-report measures are often criticized because they are subject to intentional as well as unintentional response biases. Self-reports about health-related behavior are particularly suspect because they often deal with issues that are considered to be socially sensitive—for example, use of illicit substances (Kristiansen and Harding, 1984). Despite these apparent problems, self-report measures are usually the most reliable and valid indicators that are available. In addition, because of pragmatic or ethical constraints, they are often the only measures that can be obtained (see D'Onofrio, this volume).

In an effort to enhance the validity of self-reports, special survey-administration methods have been developed, including the randomized response (Warner, 1965), the "bogus pipeline" (Evans, Hansen, and Mittelmark, 1977), and the respondent code-generated identifier techniques (Carifio and Biron, 1978). However, each of these methods has associated problems that may reduce the overall internal and external validity of an evaluation study (Nederhoff, 1984). Although numerous studies have been conducted to assess the utility of these techniques, the evidence is not consistent that any are superior to a carefully conducted, group-administered survey that stresses confidentiality in an effort to maximize respondents' trust. Furthermore, none of the methodological studies was conducted as part of a program evaluation; thus, the results may not be generalizable to evaluation studies (Malvin and Moskowitz, 1983). In an evaluation study, some degree of response bias can be tolerated as long as the amount of bias is comparable across conditions and the study's statistical power is not substantially reduced. The presence of an intervention in the program condition, however, may create greater pressures to respond in a socially desirable manner in this condition relative to the comparison condition, regardless of the procedures used to collect self-report data (Malvin and Moskowitz, 1983). This hypothesis can be tested if an alternative measure is available to validate the self-reports. Data from the self-report measure should be regressed on the alternative measure, separately for each condition and then across conditions. If the former model does not fit the data significantly better than the latter model, one can rule out differential response bias (assuming adequate variability in these measures).

Social desirability pressures are probably strongest soon after the completion of a program and diminish over time. Thus, the results from a posttest conducted at the conclusion of a program are most suspect. Fortunately, these results are usually of less interest than longer-term follow-ups, which should be less biased. It is critical to document the data collection procedures carefully because this information may ultimately be the most useful in judging response validity.

Research Design. Basic details about the research design should be presented, including when and where the study was conducted and when the measures were collected. The report should describe how subjects were assigned to conditions and when they learned what their respective conditions were (before recruitment, before or after pretest). Any matching or stratification procedures that were used should be described. If randomization was employed, were subjects or some larger social grouping (for example, schools) randomized, and when did randomization occur?

"For all types of evaluations, a clear approach or design should be specified and justified as appropriate to the types of conclusions and inferences to be drawn" (ERS Standards Committee, 1982, p. 13). Experimental designs where individual subjects are randomly assigned to conditions enable the researcher to make much stronger inferences about the effects of a program than does a quasi-experiment where assignment is not random. However, such studies may not be feasible or may not be desirable. For example, it would not make sense to assign students in the same school to experimental and control conditions when the social interactions of experimental and control students over time may influence the target behaviors. Furthermore, the policy implications of this type of study may be limited because it is unlikely that the program would ever be disseminated in this fashion. Thus, for theoretical and practical reasons, some evaluations assign larger social units to conditions (for example, schools or communities). If only a few units are randomly assigned to each condition, then the degree of initial equivalence among conditions required by a true experiment is not likely to be obtained. Furthermore, even when the conditions appear to be equivalent at pretest, the effects of local history (Cook and Campbell, 1979) are more likely to introduce bias. Ideally, a substantial number of units should be assigned to each condition. However, because of the cost and difficulty of conducting a large-scale evaluation, this is not always feasible.

"Provision should be made for the detection, reconciliation, and documentation of departures from the original design" (ERS Standards Committee, 1982, p. 14). Even a well-designed randomized field experiment may deteriorate into a quasi-experiment because of the occurrence of a variety of real-world events (for example, differential participation or attrition of subjects across conditions). Therefore, evaluation reports must provide sufficient details about the research design and local historical events to substantiate that the experimental design was maintained.

Subject Attrition. Attrition of subjects (and sometimes also social units) constitutes a serious potential threat to the internal and external validity of experimental and quasi-experimental studies. In order to determine whether subject attrition has affected the internal validity of the study, two types of analyses should be conducted. First, the rate of attrition should be analyzed by condition, to determine whether it is differential across conditions. If social units (such as schools) were assigned to condition, all subjects contained within these units at pretest who were originally eligible for the study should be used in computing attrition, not just those who completed the pretest. After all, it is just as important to determine whether initial participation in the study is biased as it is to examine subsequent participation. Second, the pattern of attrition should be analyzed by comparison of scores on all pretest measures of those who were lost to follow-up versus those who were not (attrition status) for each of the conditions (Jurs and Glass, 1971). In this analysis, a significant main effect for condition, or an interaction between attrition status and condition, provides evidence that the internal validity of the study has been compromised. This latter analysis can also indicate the extent to which the study's external validity is limited. A significant main effect for attrition status would provide evidence for limited external validity.

Statistical Analysis and Results. The ERS standards focus considerable attention on data analysis because the issues involved in analyzing outcome evaluation data are often complex: "The analytic procedures should be matched to the purposes of the evaluation, the design, and the data collection. . . . Analytic procedures should be appropriate to the properties of the measures and to the quality and quantity of the data. . . . Justification should be provided that the appropriate analytic procedures have been applied. . . . Documentation should be adequate to make the analyses replicable" (ERS Standards Committee, 1982, p. 14–15).

"For impact studies, the central evaluation design problem of estimating the effects of nontreatment and the choice of a particular method for accomplishing this should be fully described and justified" (ERS Standards Committee, 1982, p. 13). This is quite straightforward when an experimental design is employed, as long as the design did not deteriorate. Any one of a number of textbook approaches (for example, analysis of covariance) can be used to analyze the data. However, when an experimental design deteriorates or a nonequivalent comparison group is utilized, there is no single analysis that is likely to yield unbiased estimates of a program's effects (Reichardt and Gollob, 1986). The nonequivalent comparison group design is subject to numerous influences that create nonrandom as well as random sources of uncertainty when trying to attribute to the program any differences found between the conditions on the posttest measures (Reichardt, 1979). In order to understand the nature and extent of these biases, all of the pretest measures should be analyzed to determine whether conditions were different before the intervention, and any significant differences should be reported. To reduce the considerable uncertainty in estimating program effects with this design, multiple analyses should then be conducted, yielding "plausibility brackets" around the estimated program effects (Reichardt and Gollob, 1986). These analyses should make different assumptions about the nonrandom biases that operate across conditions.

"All analytic procedures, along with their underlying assumptions and limitations, should be described explicitly, and the reasons for choosing the procedures should be clearly explained" (ERS Standards Committee, 1982, p. 15). The assumptions underlying the statistical models selected must be tested using available data. This is essential because data from evaluation studies often violate multiple assumptions of commonly used analyses. For example, analyses based on ordinary least-squares estimation (such as multiple regression or analysis of variance and covariance) are not robust to violations of homogeneity of variance and covariance or independence of observations. Conducting these analyses when major assumptions are violated yields results that are uninterpretable: Tests of significance are spurious, and estimates of program effects are biased.

Statistical power, or the likelihood that the research design can detect a real program effect of a reasonable magnitude, should be discussed. This is particularly important when a study fails to find significant effects on one of the major dependent variables. Evaluations of treatment interventions typically have had inadequate statistical power because of the small sample sizes utilized in these studies (Lipsey, 1988). Prevention program evaluations usually do not suffer from this problem because sample sizes are often in the hundreds or thousands. For other reasons, however, statistical power is often problematic in prevention studies.

First, because only a small portion of the target population is at risk for the health-compromising behavior, small program effects are likely to have practical significance. Thus, prevention studies should be designed with sufficient power to detect small effects. In some instances, it may be warranted to increase the statistical power of a study by increasing the Type I error rate—from the conventional .05 level, for example, to .10. Second, prevention studies typically require long-term follow-up in order to demonstrate effectiveness or to demonstrate that an effect is sustained long enough to be meaningful. The research design must make accommodations to the decreased statistical power because of the sheer number of subjects lost over time and the likelihood that many of the high-risk subjects will be lost.

"The units of analysis should be appropriate to the way the data were collected and the types of conclusions to be drawn" (ERS Standards Committee, 1982, p. 14). Although it may be more appropriate to analyze the units that were assigned to condition (that is, the subjects' data could be aggregated within social units before analysis) or to conduct a multilevel analysis, this is often not done because statistical power may be inadequate, given the small number of units employed. However, analysis of individual subjects' data that does not take the multilevel nature of a design into account is likely to violate the assumption that observations are independent and is liable to yield results that are meaningless (see Koepke and Flay, this volume).

Discussion

The discussion section of an evaluation report should "examine, interpret, and qualify the results, as well as to draw inferences from them" (American Psychological Association, 1986, p. 27). The implications of the findings for the program theory and the process implementation theory should be addressed. If the program as delivered deviated from the program as designed, the reasons for these deviations should be discussed, as well as the implications for refinement and dissemination of the program.

The "findings should be reported in a manner that distinguishes among objective findings, opinions, judgments, and speculation" (ERS Standards Committee, 1982, p. 15). The authors of a report should not assume that readers can critically evaluate the study's methodology, for evaluation reports are often read by audiences in search of a program who lack research training. In fact, many readers may only examine the report's abstract or its introduction and its discussion section. Thus, it is imperative that authors provide an objective interpretation of the facts and present the appropriate caveats about the study's implications. Any features of the study that may have substantially influenced the study's findings should be discussed.

"Cause-and-effect interpretations should be bolstered not only by reference to the design but also by recognition and elimination of plausible rival explanations" (ERS Standards Committee, 1982, p. 15). Because the researchers are closest to the data, they are likely to have considerable insight into plausible alternative hypotheses for the study's findings. As scientists, the researchers are obligated to raise these hypotheses, especially ones that cannot be summarily rejected. Naturally, if explanations can be ruled out through additional data analysis, then the appropriate analysis should be conducted.

"When quantitative comparisons are made, indications should be provided of both statistical and practical significance" (ERS Standards Committee, 1982, p. 15). That an effect has obtained statistical significance does not ensure that it is practically significant. Factors that help determine whether an effect has practical significance may include the magnitude and duration of the effect, the subgroups for which the effect was obtained, and the social and economic costs of delivering the program relative to the costs of the problem that is prevented.

"There is rather substantial agreement that the more independent the evaluator is, the more credible the results of the impact evaluation will be. . . . Potential conflicts of interest should be identified, and steps should be taken to avoid compromising the evaluation processes and results" (ERS Standards Committee, 1982, pp. 10, 12). When real or apparent conflicts of interest exist among researchers or their organization and the program under evaluation, the research report should document the nature of these relationships, as well as any precautions taken to prevent bias.

Conclusion

This chapter proposes a preliminary set of guidelines for reporting outcome evaluation studies of health promotion and disease prevention programs. Because few studies will be able to overcome all potential threats to validity, it is essential that research be reported in a comprehensive manner so that a scientifically based literature can evolve.

Although this chapter focuses on technical issues that commonly detract from the interpretability of outcome evaluation studies, I believe that many of the shortcomings identified here are not simply due to technical problems. If this is true, disseminating more specific research guidelines will not be sufficient to promote better research. Therefore, in a subsequent work, I will examine institutional pressures and barriers that act as disincentives to the conduct of better outcome evaluation research, and I will propose remedies for these problems (Moskowitz, in preparation).

References

American Psychological Association. *Publication Manual of the American Psychological Association.* (3rd ed.) Washington, D.C.: American Psychological Association, 1986.

Bickman, L. (ed.). *Using Program Theory in Evaluation.* New Directions for Program Evaluation, no. 33. San Francisco: Jossey-Bass, 1987.

Boruch, R., and Gomez, H. "Sensitivity, Bias, and Theory in Impact Evaluations." In L. Sechrest and others (eds.), *Evaluation Studies Review Annual.* Vol. 4. Newbury Park, Calif.: Sage, 1979.

✗ Bruvold, W. H., and Rundall, T. G. "A Meta-Analysis and Theoretical Review of School Based Tobacco and Alcohol Intervention Programs." *Psychology and Health,* 1988, *2,* 53-78.

Carifio, J., and Biron, R. "Collecting Sensitive Data Anonymously: The CDRGP Technique." *Journal of Alcohol and Drug Education,* 1978, *23,* 47-66.

Chalmers, T., Smith, H., Blackburn, B., Silverman, B., Schroeder, B., Reitman, D., and Ambroz, A. "A Method for Assessing the Quality of a Randomized Control Trial." *Controlled Clinical Trials,* 1981, *2,* 31-49.

Cook, T. D., and Campbell, D. T. *Quasi-Experimentation: Design and Analysis Issues for Field Settings.* Skokie, Ill.: Rand McNally, 1979.

ERS Standards Committee. "Evaluation Research Society Standards for Program Evaluation." In P. H. Rossi (ed.), *Standards for Evaluation Practice.* New Directions for Program Evaluation, no. 15. San Francisco: Jossey-Bass, 1982.

Evans, R. I., Hansen, W., and Mittelmark, M. "Increasing the Validity of Self-Reports of Smoking Behavior in Children." *Journal of Applied Psychology,* 1977, *62,* 521-523.

Flay, B. "Psychosocial Approaches to Smoking Prevention: A Review of Findings." *Health Psychology,* 1985, *4,* 449-488.

Joint Committee on Standards for Educational Evaluation. *Standards for Evaluations of Educational Programs, Projects, and Materials.* New York: McGraw-Hill, 1981.

Judd, C., and Kenny, D. "Process Analysis: Estimating Mediation in Treatment Evaluations." *Evaluation Review,* 1981, *5,* 602-619.

Jurs, S., and Glass, G. "The Effect of Experimental Mortality on the Internal and External Validity of the Randomized Comparative Experiment." *Journal of Experimental Education,* 1971, *40,* 62-66.

Kristiansen, C., and Harding, C. "The Social Desirability of Preventive Health Behavior." *Public Health Reports,* 1984, *99* (4), 384-388.

Lipsey, M. W. "Practice and Malpractice in Evaluation Research." *Evaluation Practice,* 1988, *9* (4), 5-24.

Malvin, J., and Moskowitz, J. "Anonymous Versus Identifiable Self-Reports of Adolescent Drug Attitudes, Intentions, and Use." *Public Opinion Quarterly,* 1983, *47,* 557-566.

Moskowitz, J. "The Primary Prevention of Alcohol Problems: A Critical Review of the Research Literature." *Journal of Studies on Alcohol,* 1989, *50,* 54-88.

Moskowitz, J. *Why Outcome Evaluations Are Uninterpretable: Issues and Possible Solutions.* Berkeley: School of Public Health, University of California, in press.

Mosteller, F., Gilbert, J., and McPeek, B. "Reporting Standards and Research Strategies for Controlled Trials: Agenda for the Editor." *Controlled Clinical Trials,* 1980, *1,* 37-58.

Nederhoff, A. "Methods of Coping with Social Desirability Bias: A Review." *European Journal of Social Psychology*, 1984, *15*, 263–280.

Office for Substance Abuse Prevention. *Demonstration Grants for the Prevention, Treatment, and Rehabilitation of Drug and Alcohol Abuse Among High-Risk Youth.* Request for Applications (AD 89-03). Rockville, Md.: Alcohol, Drug Abuse, and Mental Health Administration, Department of Health and Human Services, 1989.

Patton, M. "Evaluation of Program Implementation." *Evaluation Studies Review Annual*, 1979, *4*, 318–346.

Reichardt, C. "The Statistical Analysis of Data from Nonequivalent Group Designs." In T. D. Cook and D. T. Campbell (eds.), *Quasi-Experimentation: Design and Analysis Issues for Field Settings.* Skokie, Ill.: Rand McNally, 1979.

Reichardt, C., and Gollob, H. "Taking Uncertainty into Account When Estimating Effects." In W.M.K. Trochim (ed.), *Advances in Quasi-Experimental Design and Analysis.* New Directions for Program Evaluation, no. 31. San Francisco: Jossey-Bass, 1986.

Riecken, H., and Boruch, R. *Social Experimentation: A Method for Planning and Evaluating Social Intervention.* Orlando, Fla.: Academic Press, 1974.

Rothman, A., and Byrne, N. "Health Education for Children and Adolescents." *Review of Educational Research*, 1981, *51*, 85–100.

Schaps, E., DiBartolo, R., Moskowitz, J., Palley, C., and Churgin, S. "Primary Prevention Evaluation Research: A Review of 127 Impact Studies." *Journal of Drug Issues*, 1981, *11*, 17–43.

Warner, S. L. "Randomized Response: A Survey Technique for Eliminating Evasive Answer Bias." *Journal of the American Statistical Association*, 1965, *60*, 63–69.

Joel M. Moskowitz is adjunct associate professor and associate research psychologist in the School of Public Health at the University of California, Berkeley. His research focuses on preventing abuse of tobacco, alcohol, and other substances. He currently serves on a National Institute on Drug Abuse committee that reviews grant applications for epidemiology and prevention research.

Index